Neisseria gonorrhoeae Infections

Neisseria gonorrhoeae Infections

Editors

María-Teresa Pérez-Gracia
Beatriz Suay-García

MDPI • Basel • Beijing • Wuhan • Barcelona • Belgrade • Manchester • Tokyo • Cluj • Tianjin

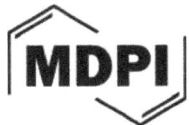

Editors
María-Teresa Pérez-Gracia
Universidad Cardenal Herrera-CEU,
CEU Universities
Spain

Beatriz Suay-García
Universidad Cardenal Herrera-CEU,
CEU Universities
Spain

Editorial Office
MDPI
St. Alban-Anlage 66
4052 Basel, Switzerland

This is a reprint of articles from the Special Issue published online in the open access journal *Pathogens* (ISSN 2076-0817) (available at: https://www.mdpi.com/journal/pathogens/special_issues/Neisseria_gonorrhoeae_Infections).

For citation purposes, cite each article independently as indicated on the article page online and as indicated below:

LastName, A.A.; LastName, B.B.; LastName, C.C. Article Title. *Journal Name* **Year**, *Volume Number*, Page Range.

ISBN 978-3-0365-0790-3 (Hbk)
ISBN 978-3-0365-0791-0 (PDF)

© 2021 by the authors. Articles in this book are Open Access and distributed under the Creative Commons Attribution (CC BY) license, which allows users to download, copy and build upon published articles, as long as the author and publisher are properly credited, which ensures maximum dissemination and a wider impact of our publications.

The book as a whole is distributed by MDPI under the terms and conditions of the Creative Commons license CC BY-NC-ND.

Contents

About the Editors vii

Beatriz Suay-García and María-Teresa Pérez-Gracia
Neisseria gonorrhoeae Infections
Reprinted from: *Pathogens* **2020**, *9*, 647, doi:10.3390/pathogens9080647 1

Susu M. Zughaier, Corinne E. Rouquette-Loughlin and William M. Shafer
Identification of a *Neisseria gonorrhoeae* Histone Deacetylase: Epigenetic Impact on Host Gene Expression
Reprinted from: *Pathogens* **2020**, *9*, 132, doi:10.3390/pathogens9020132 5

Johan H. Melendez, Yu-Hsiang Hsieh, Mathilda Barnes, Justin Hardick,
Elizabeth A. Gilliams and Charlotte A. Gaydos
Can Ciprofloxacin be Used for Precision Treatment of Gonorrhea in Public STD Clinics? Assessment of Ciprofloxacin Susceptibility and an Opportunity for Point-of-Care Testing
Reprinted from: *Pathogens* **2019**, *8*, 189, doi:10.3390/pathogens8040189 21

Chris Kenyon
To What Extent Should We Rely on Antibiotics to Reduce High Gonococcal Prevalence? Historical Insights from Mass-Meningococcal Campaigns
Reprinted from: *Pathogens* **2020**, *9*, 134, doi:10.3390/pathogens9020134 29

Thomas Meyer and Susanne Buder
The Laboratory Diagnosis of *Neisseria gonorrhoeae*: Current Testing and Future Demands
Reprinted from: *Pathogens* **2020**, *9*, 91, doi:10.3390/pathogens9020091 37

Maria Victoria Humbert and Myron Christodoulides
Atypical, Yet Not Infrequent, Infections with *Neisseria* Species
Reprinted from: *Pathogens* **2020**, *9*, 10, doi:10.3390/pathogens9010010 57

Christophe Van Dijck, Jolein G.E. Laumen, Achilleas Tsoumanis,
Sheeba S. Manoharan-Basil and Chris Kenyon
Commensal *Neisseria* Are Shared between Sexual Partners: Implications for Gonococcal and Meningococcal Antimicrobial Resistance
Reprinted from: *Pathogens* **2020**, *9*, 228, doi:10.3390/pathogens9030228 85

About the Editors

María-Teresa Pérez-Gracia (PhD). She is currently a Full Professor of Microbiology at the CEU Cardenal Herrera University (Valencia, Spain). She holds a PhD degree with distinction in Biological Sciences from the University of Santiago de Compostela and she is a specialist in microbiology and parasitology. She has been Associate Professor of Microbiology at the Faculty of Medicine of the University of Cádiz, collaborating in research and diagnostic tasks in the Microbiology Service and in the Research Unit of the University Hospital of Puerto Real (Cádiz). She was responsible for the doctorate course "Bacterial Resistance to Antimicrobials" of the CEU Cardenal Herrera University. Currently, she directs a research line called "Molecular Diagnosis in Clinical Microbiology" on the study and detection of antimicrobial-resistant bacteria and its implications in public health, and the development and implementation of new molecular diagnostic techniques. She has received several awards, among which are the "CÁDIZ" Prize of the Royal Academy of Medicine and Surgery of Cádiz and the Angel Herrera Award for the best teaching work in the Faculty of Experimental Sciences and Health. She collaborates in the Doctorate Program "Cellular and molecular bases of human pathology" in the University of Cádiz. She was coordinator of the Advanced Specialization Degree in Clinical Analysis. She is an evaluator of projects belonging to the area of Clinical Sciences and Public Health of the Fund for Scientific and Technological Research (FONCYT) of the National Agency for Scientific and Technological Promotion (ANPCYT) of the Ministry of Science, Technology and Productive Innovation (Argentine Republic), of the General Directorate of Scientific Research and Innovation in Health of the Ministry of Health (Italy), of the National Science Centre in Physical Sciences and Engineering (Poland), the HORIZON 2020 FET-OPEN-NOVEL IDEAS FOR RADICALLY NEW TECHNOLOGIES, Research and Innovation Actions (RIA) (European Commission) and of the National Biopharma Mission Program Biotechnology Industry Research Assistance Council (BIRAC) (Government of India). She belongs to the editorial committees of several international journals and is a reviewer of scientific articles for more than 50 international journals. She is a corresponding academician at the Royal Academy of Medicine and Surgery of Cádiz and a member of the Spanish Society of Infectious Diseases and Clinical Microbiology (SEIMC) and Spanish Society of Microbiology (SEM).

Beatriz Suay-Garcia (PhD). She is currently is a research assistant at the CEU Cardenal Herrera University (Valencia, Spain). She holds a PhD degree with distinction in Pharmacy from the CEU Cardenal Herrera University. Her research is focused on antibiotic-resistant bacteria and antibiotic development.

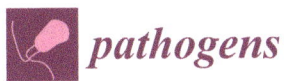

Editorial

Neisseria gonorrhoeae Infections

Beatriz Suay-García [1] and María-Teresa Pérez-Gracia [2,*]

1. ESI International Chair@CEU-UCH, Departamento de Matemáticas, Física y Ciencias Tecnológicas, Universidad Cardenal Herrera-CEU, CEU Universities, San Bartolomé 55, 46115 Alfara del Patriarca (Valencia), Spain; beatriz.suay@uchceu.es
2. Área de Microbiología. Departamento de Farmacia, Universidad Cardenal Herrera-CEU, CEU Universities, C/Ramón y Cajal s/n, 46115 Alfara del Patriarca (Valencia), Spain
* Correspondence: teresa@uchceu.es; Tel.: +34-961-369-000 (ext. 64332)

Received: 10 August 2020; Accepted: 10 August 2020; Published: 12 August 2020

Abstract: Gonorrhea is a sexually transmitted disease with a high morbidity burden. Despite having guidelines for its treatment, the incidence of the disease follows an increasing trend worldwide. This is mainly due to the appearance of antibiotic-resistant strains, inefficient diagnostic methods and poor sexual education. Without an effective vaccine available, the key priorities for the control of the disease include sexual education, contact notification, epidemiological surveillance, diagnosis and effective antibiotic treatment. This Special Issue focuses on some of these important issues such as the molecular mechanisms of the disease, diagnostic tests and different treatment strategies to combat gonorrhea.

Keywords: *Neisseria gonorrhoeae*; sexually transmitted infection; transmission; diagnosis; antibiotic treatment

---

Neisseria gonorrhoeae is an obligate human pathogen that causes gonorrhea, a sexually transmitted disease (STD). This Gram-negative diplococcus is highly infective due to its virulence factors: pili, Por proteins, Opa proteins, Rmp proteins, lipooligosaccharides and IgA protease. The most common form of presentation in men is acute anterior urethritis, while gonococcal infection in women does not have specific symptoms. Although the prevailing view is that infections in women are mainly asymptomatic whereas infections in men are not, many studies show that asymptomatic infections are prevalent in both sexes. Gonorrhea is primarily transmitted from an infected individual by direct human-to-human contact between the mucosal membranes of the urogenital tract, anal canal and the oropharynx, usually during sexual activities.

Gonorrhea is a community disease with a high morbidity burden, representing 88 million of the estimated 448 million new cases of curable STDs that occur yearly worldwide [1]. Furthermore, the incidence of the disease is rising due to the prevalence of multidrug-resistant strains [2]. In fact, the appearance of resistances in this microorganism threatens the effectiveness of the available gonorrhea treatments to such extent that it has been classified as a "Priority 2" microorganism in the WHO *Global Priority List of Antibiotic-Resistant Bacteria to Guide Research, Discovery, and Development of New Antibiotics* [3]. Ever since sulphonamides were introduced to treat gonorrhea in the 1930s, gonococci have continuously shown an extraordinary ability to develop resistance to any antimicrobial introduced for treatment [4]. Treatment is currently given empirically, without performing antimicrobial susceptibility tests. However, the increasing issue of drug-resistant gonococci has led the scientific community to focus research on new drugs and alternative treatments, which has obtained encouraging results. The diagnosis of gonorrhea is established by identification of *N. gonorrhoeae* in genital, rectal, pharyngeal or ocular secretions. *N. gonorrhoeae* can be detected by culture or nucleic acid amplification tests and, in some cases, Gram staining. Without an effective vaccine available, the key priorities for the prevention and control of the disease include public health and sexual education, contact notification, epidemiological surveillance, early diagnosis and effective antibiotic treatment.

In this Special Issue, which is devoted to understanding some of the important issues about *Neisseria gonorrhoeae* infection, there are six contributions in the form of original research papers, review articles and a brief report focused on the physiopathology of gonorrhea, diagnostic tests and different treatment strategies against this STD. More specifically, the first research article focuses on the identification of an *N. gonorrhoeae* histone deacetylase [5]. The research conducted shows that the presence of this enzyme during gonococcal infection reduces the expression of host defense peptides and stimulates promoters of pro-inflammatory mediator genes. These discoveries suggest that gonococci can exert epigenetic modifications on host cells to modulate macrophage defense genes, leading to a poorer trained immunity response.

The second research article assesses ciprofloxacin susceptibility in strains obtained from patients attending STD clinics to receive treatment [6]. The strains isolated in STD clinics in Baltimore (USA) had an overall ciprofloxacin resistance prevalence of 32.4% when evaluated by Gyrase A PCR and E-test. It must be noted that this percentage increased over the years studied, from an initial 24.7% in 2014 to 45.2% in 2016. Researchers conclude that, in this environment, ciprofloxacin could be used as a targeted treatment. However, they highlight that point-of-care tests for *N. gonorrhoeae* diagnosis and susceptibility testing are urgently needed to identify individuals who can be treated with this targeted approach.

Furthermore, three insightful review articles discuss relevant topics such as the assessment of the risks of relying on antibiotics to reduce gonococcal prevalence by analyzing historical data on the appearance of antibiotic resistance after mass-meningococcal campaigns [7]; the different laboratory diagnostic options available and future options for a more efficient and affordable diagnosis [8]; and the diversity of the genus *Neisseria* in the clinical context, bringing attention to the many pathologies these species may cause [9]. Lastly, a brief report analyzes the transmission of commensal *Neisseria* between sexual partners and the implications this may have in the transmission of antibacterial resistances [10].

Author Contributions: Both authors, B.S.-G. and M.-T.P.-G., contributed equally in the writing of this article, including conceptualization, writing, reviewing and editing. All authors have read and agreed to the published version of the manuscript.

Funding: This research received no external funding.

Conflicts of Interest: The authors declare no conflict of interest.

References

1. WHO. Emergence of Multi-Drug Resistant *Neisseria gonorrhoeae*—Threat of Global Rise in Untreatable Sexually Transmitted Infections (Fact Sheet). Available online: https://www.who.int/reproductivehealth/publications/rtis/who_rhr_11_14/en/ (accessed on 4 August 2020).
2. Unemo, M.; Seifert, H.S.; Hook, E.W.; Hawkes, S.; Ndowa, F.; Dillon, J.-A.R. Gonorrhoea. *Nat. Rev. Dis. Primers.* **2019**, *5*, 79. [PubMed]
3. WHO. Global Priority List of Antibiotic-Resistant Bacteria to Guide Research, Discovery, and Development of New Antibiotics. Available online: https://www.who.int/medicines/publications/WHO-PPL-Short_Summary_25Feb-ET_NM_WHO.pdf?ua=1 (accessed on 4 August 2020).
4. Suay-García, B.; Pérez-Gracia, M.T. Future Prospects for *Neisseria gonorrhoeae* Treatment. *Antibiotics* **2018**, *7*, 49. [CrossRef] [PubMed]
5. Zughaier, S.M.; Rouquette-Loughlin, C.E.; Shafer, W.M. Identification of a *Neisseria gonorrhoeae* Histone Deacetylase: Epigenetic Impact on Host Gene Expression. *Pathogens* **2020**, *9*, 132. [CrossRef] [PubMed]
6. Melendez, J.H.; Hsieh, Y.-H.; Barnes, M.; Hardick, J.; Gilliams, E.A.; Gaydos, C.A. Can Ciprofloxacin be Used for Precision Treatment of Gonorrhea in Public STD Clinics? Assessment of Ciprofloxacin Susceptibility and an Opportunity for Point-of-Care Testing. *Pathogens* **2019**, *8*, 189. [CrossRef] [PubMed]
7. Kenyon, C. To What Extent Should We Rely on Antibiotics to Reduce High Gonococcal Prevalence? Historical Insights from Mass-Meningococcal Campaigns. *Pathogens* **2020**, *9*, 134. [CrossRef] [PubMed]

8. Meyer, T.; Buder, S. The Laboratory Diagnosis of *Neisseria gonorrhoeae*: Current Testing and Future Demands. *Pathogens* **2020**, *9*, 91. [CrossRef] [PubMed]
9. Humbert, M.V.; Christodoulides, M. Atypical, Yet Not Infrequent, Infections with *Neisseria* Species. *Pathogens* **2020**, *9*, 10. [CrossRef] [PubMed]
10. Van Dijck, C.; Laumen, J.G.E.; Manoharan-Basil, S.S.; Kenyon, C. Commensal *Neisseria* Are Shared between Sexual Partners: Implications for Gonococcal and Meningococcal Antimicrobial Resistance. *Pathogens* **2020**, *9*, 228. [CrossRef] [PubMed]

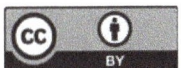

© 2020 by the authors. Licensee MDPI, Basel, Switzerland. This article is an open access article distributed under the terms and conditions of the Creative Commons Attribution (CC BY) license (http://creativecommons.org/licenses/by/4.0/).

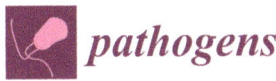

Article

Identification of a *Neisseria gonorrhoeae* Histone Deacetylase: Epigenetic Impact on Host Gene Expression

Susu M. Zughaier [1,*], Corinne E. Rouquette-Loughlin [2,3] and William M. Shafer [2,3,4]

1. Department of Basic Medical Sciences, College of Medicine, QU Health, Qatar University, P.O. Box 2713, Doha, Qatar
2. Laboratory of Bacterial Pathogenesis, Department of Veterans Affairs Medical Center, Decatur, GA 30033, USA; corinne@patweb.com (C.E.R.-L.); wshafer@emory.edu (W.M.S.)
3. Department of Microbiology and Immunology, Emory University School of Medicine, Atlanta, GA 30322, USA
4. The Emory Antibiotic Research Center, Emory University School of Medicine, Atlanta, GA 30322, USA
* Correspondence: szughaier@qu.edu.qa; Tel.: +974-4403-7859

Received: 14 January 2020; Accepted: 14 February 2020; Published: 18 February 2020

Abstract: Epigenetic reprogramming in macrophages is termed trained innate immunity, which regulates immune tolerance and limits tissue damage during infection. *Neisseria gonorrhoeae* is a strict human pathogen that causes the sexually transmitted infection termed gonorrhea. Here, we report that this pathogen harbors a gene that encodes a histone deacetylase-like enzyme (Gc-HDAC) that shares high 3D-homology to human HDAC1, HDAC2 and HDAC8. A Gc-HDAC null mutant was constructed to determine the biologic significance of this gene. The results showed that WT gonococci reduced the expression of host defense peptides LL-37, HBD-1 and SLPI in macrophages when compared to its Gc-HDAC-deficient isogenic strain. The enrichment of epigenetic marks in histone tails control gene expression and are known to change during bacterial infections. To investigate whether gonococci exert epigenetic modifications on host chromatin, the enrichment of acetylated lysine 9 in histone 3 (H3K9ac) was investigated using the TLR-focused ChIP array system. The data showed that infection with WT gonococci led to higher H3K9ac enrichment at the promoters of pro-inflammatory mediators' genes, many TLRs, adaptor proteins and transcription factors, suggesting gene activation when compared to infection with the Gc-HDAC-deficient mutant. Taken together, the data suggest that gonococci can exert epigenetic modifications on host cells to modulate certain macrophage defense genes, leading to a maladaptive state of trained immunity.

Keywords: *Neisseria gonorrhoeae*; HDAC; infection; epigenetic; H3K9ac; macrophage; survival; cytokines; chemokines; gonorrhea

---

1. Introduction

Neisseria gonorrhoeae is a strict human pathogen that causes the sexually transmitted infection termed gonorrhea. Importantly, gonorrhea is a major worldwide public health problem given its estimated yearly incidence of 87 million infections [1]. In addition to causing a high incidence of infection and disease, the gonococcus is noted for its capacity to develop resistance to antibiotics used in therapy [1]. In 2013, the Center for Disease Control declared antibiotic-resistant *N. gonorrhoeae* as an urgent threat to public health [2–4]. Recently, the World Health Organization placed *N. gonorrhoeae* on the high priority pathogen list for developing new antibiotics [5,6].

Gonococci can survive extracellularly and intracellularly, but, in both environments, the bacteria must adapt to pressures exerted by the host [7,8]. We reported that *N. gonorrhoeae* can survive in association with human monocytes and murine macrophages [9]. During infection of these phagocytes, it was noted that gonococci can enhance expression of iron-responsive genes encoding hepcidin (a master iron-regulating hormone), the antimicrobial protein termed NGAL and NRAMP1 while downregulating expression of the gene encoding the short chain 3-hydroxybutyrate dehydrogenase (BDH2) that catalyzes the production of the mammalian siderophore 2,5-DHBA involved in chelating and detoxifying iron. Based on these findings, we proposed that N. gonorrhoeae can subvert the iron-limiting innate immune defenses to facilitate iron acquisition and intracellular survival [7].

N. gonorrhoeae possesses several virulence factors that facilitate invasion and infection in human host. The addition of phosphoethanolamine (PEA) to lipid A by the enzyme PEA trasnferase, encoded by the phase-variable *lptA* gene [10], is important for bacterial resistance to cationic antimicrobial peptides [11] and complement-mediated killing by normal human serum [10,12]. PEA modification on lipid A enhanced bacterial survival within human polymorphonuclear leukocytes [13] and increased fitness of gonococci during experimental lower genital tract infection of female mice or in the urethra of human male volunteers [14,15]. Further, we recently reported that this PEA modification of lipid A reduced autophagy flux in macrophages, consequently delaying bacterial clearance and promoting intracellular survival [9]. Taken together, PEA-lipid A modification is a critical component in the ability of *N. gonorrhoeae* to evade host defenses and survive in macrophages.

The ability of gonococci to develop resistance to host AMPs prompted us to determine if this human pathogen might also modulate their production by phagocytes. In this respect, a previous report documented that live gonococci can downregulate cervical epithelial cell production of LL-37, a potent anti-gonococcal CAMP also produced by macrophages/monocytes and PMNs, to facilitate host cell invasion [16]. However, the mechanism by which gonococci downregulate host AMPs is unknown.

In order to explore the mechanism of *CAMP* gene suppression, we evaluated the potential impact of epigenetic factors. Although studies with other bacterial pathogens have documented the role of epigenetic factors, including histone deacetylases, it was heretofore unknown if gonococci can exert epigenetic modifications on host histones, thereby modulating host gene expression. Histones are highly basic proteins found in all eukaryotic cells and are required for packaging DNA in chromatin structures. Core histones have long tails that protrude from the nucleosome, which are targets for posttranslational modifications that consequently alter their interaction with DNA and nuclear proteins. Histone tail modifications include acetylation, methylation, phosphorylation, uniquitination, SUMOylation, citrullination and ADP-ribosylation [17]. These modifications influence various biological processes involved in DNA repair, gene regulation and cell division [17]. Several enzymes are involved in histone epigenetic modifications, including histone methyltranferases (HMT), histone acetyl transferases (HAT) and histone deacetylase (HDAC). The degree of lysine acetylation in core histone tails in particular directly influence transcriptional regulation, since acetylation reduces the positive charge on lysine, leading to reduced binding to the negatively charged DNA, thereby loosening chromatin structures facilitating transcription factors (TFs) binding to gene promoters. In contrast, deacetylation of lysine residues by HDACs increases the positive charges on histone tails that tighten its binding to DNA, rendering TFs binding sites inaccessible, resulting in gene suppression [18,19]. Against this background, we now report that gonococci (as well as commensal *Neisseria*) encode a highly conserved HDAC-like protein, herein named Gc-HDAC, that shares very high 3D homology to human HDAC1, HDAC2 and HDAC8. However, the function of this Gc-HDAC-like enzyme in gonococci is not known. We hypothesized that the Gc-HDAC-like protein exerts epigenetic modifications on host histones to suppress LL-37 and HBD-1 gene expression, which facilitates immune evasion and promotes intracellular survival. In this respect, we found that *N. gonorrhoeae* can exert epigenetic modifications on host chromatin where the epigenetic mark H3K9ac is highly enriched at the promoters of certain proinflammatory genes.

2. Results

2.1. Gonococcal Infection Downregulates Host Defense Peptides Expression in Macrophages

We previously reported that *Neisseria gonorrhoeae* survives in macrophages and induces robust cytokine and chemokine release [7]. In addition to its capacity to resist the action of antibacterial agents, including AMPs, we hypothesized that gonococci could influence expression of genes encoding host defensive responses. In support of this hypothesis, a previous report showed that gonococci can downregulate the expression of the human host defense AMP LL-37 in cervical epithelial cells for immune evasion [16]. Accordingly, in order to learn if gonococci could influence expression of host genes involved in innate immunity, we first investigated the expression of human AMPs LL-37, HBD1 and SLPI in THP-1 macrophage-like monocytic cells infected with live gonococcal strain FA19. The data demonstrated that gonococcal infection led to significant reduction in the expression of LL-37, HBD1 and SLPI compared to uninfected cells using quantitative RT-PCR (Figure 1A). We also investigated the expression of LL-37 in primary human peripheral monocytes obtained from healthy donors. We found that live gonococcal infection in primary human monocytes significantly reduced the expression of LL-37 when compared to uninfected cells (Figure 1B). Further, gonococcal infection also reduced LL-37 expression of human THP-1 cells, even when this gene was overexpressed by the addition of 10 nM of 1,25-dihydroxy vitamin D3, the active form of vitamin D3 (Figure 1C). Taken together, the data suggest that gonococcal infection of human macrophages can modulate host defense peptide expression. As will be described below, expression of host genes encoding cytokines and chemokines involved in innate host response to gonococcal infection can also be influenced by gonococci during infection.

2.2. Neisseria Gonorrhoeae Contains a Gene Encoding a Histone Deacetylase-Like (Gc-HDAC) Enzyme

We hypothesized that the significant reduction in LL-37 gene expression in macrophages infected with live gonococci could be related to epigenetic modifications at the promoter of LL-37, resulting in decreased expression of the cognate gene. Accordingly, we performed a bioinformatics analysis of whole genome sequences from pathogenic and nonpathogenic *Neisseria spp.* searching for bacterial homologs of epigenetic modifying genes. Through this analysis, we detected an open reading frame (ORF) that could encode an HDAC-like enzyme. This ORF (termed *hdac*) was found in all pathogenic (*N. gonorrhoeae* and *N. meningitidis*) and commensal *Neisseria* species (*N. cinerea, N. lactamica, N. subflava, N. flavescens, N. sicca* and *N. elongata*); in gonococci, the ORF had been assigned NGO0187 in strain FA1090; NGEG_0305 in strain FA19 and NGK_0316 in strain NCCP11945 (https://blast.ncbi.nlm.nih.gov/Blast.cgi, https://www.kegg.jp/dbget-bin/www_bget?ngo:NGO0187 and https://www.genome.jp/dbget-bin/www_bget?ngk:NGK_0316, respectively). We termed the ORF as *hdac* as it is predicted to encode a highly conserved HDAC-like protein that shares 3D homology to human HDAC1, HDAC2 and HDAC8 (Figure 2). Currently, a total of 476 sequenced *Neisseria gonorrhoeae* strains have been found to contain this histone deacetylase protein homolog, which is reflected in the NCBI protein search (https://www.ncbi.nlm.nih.gov/protein).

2.3. Computational Analysis of Gc-HDAC Enzyme

Computational analysis was performed on Gc-HDAC from gonococcal strains FA19, FA1090, MS11 and GD12. Computational modeling revealed that the protein has an active catalytic pocket containing the highly conserved zinc-binding triad (Asp185, His187 and Asp268) and shares high 3D homology to human HDAC1, HDAC2 and HDAC8 [20,21] and to bacterial HDLP from *Aquifex* and *Bordetella* [22]. Although the Gc-HDAC-like protein amino acid sequence homology to human and bacterial counterparts is relatively low (HDAC1 is 22%, HDAC2 is 19%, to human HDAC8 is 20% and to bacterial HDLPs is 29% and 30%, respectively), their 3D structural homology is remarkably high (Figure 3A). Furthermore, computational docking analysis using I-TASSER predicted that several HDAC inhibitors, such as trichostatin A (TSA); CF3 (9,9,9-trifluoro-8-oxo-N-phenylnonanamide); a fluorinated analog of SAHA; CRI (5-(4-methyl-benzoylamino)-biphenyl-3,4'-dicarboxylic acid 3-dimethylamide-4'-hydroxyamide) (Figure 3B) and B3N, also called M344 (4-(dimethylamino)-N-[7-(hydroxyamino)-7-oxoheptyl]benzamide), are able to bind to the catalytic core of the enzyme (Figure 3B). HDAC inhibitors compound structures are available at https://pubchem.ncbi.nlm.nih.gov/compound.

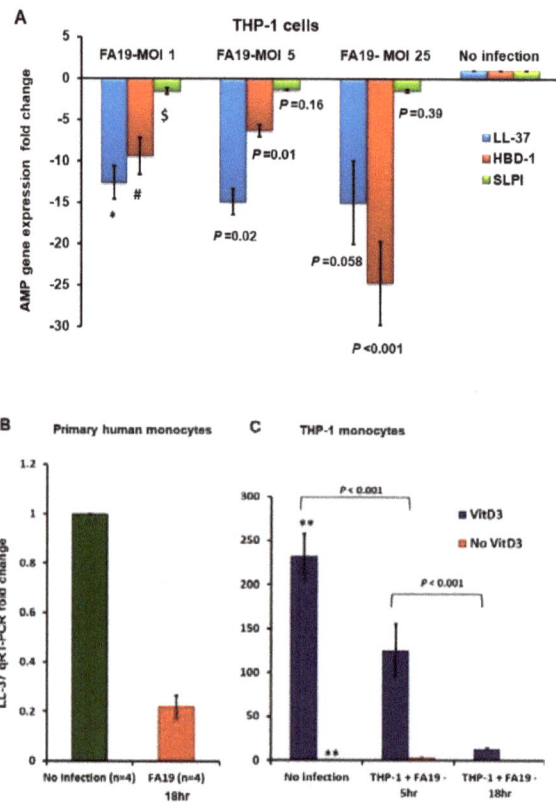

Figure 1. Gonococcal infection downregulates LL-37 and HBD-1 expression in monocytes. (**A**): Antimicrobial host defense peptide (AMP) gene expression in THP-1 cells infected with Gc strain FA19 overnight at multiplicity of infection (MOI) of 1, 5 and 25 measured by qRT-PCR. (**B**): LL-37 gene expression in primary human monocytes infected with Gc strain FA19 overnight at MOI of 10 measured by qRT-PCR. Peripheral monocytes were obtained from four different healthy donors. (**C**): Overexpression of LL-37 gene in human THP-1 monocytes treated with 10 nM of 1,25 dihydroxyvitamin D3 (VitD3) overnight prior to infection with Gc strain FA19 at MOI of 25. Downregulation of LL-37 gene expression was assessed at 5h and 18h post-infection. p values were calculated using a Student's t-test in reference to noninfected cells (**). p values in reference to infection at MOI 1 for LL-37 expression (*), HBD1 (#) and SLPI ($). These data are representative of three independent experiments.

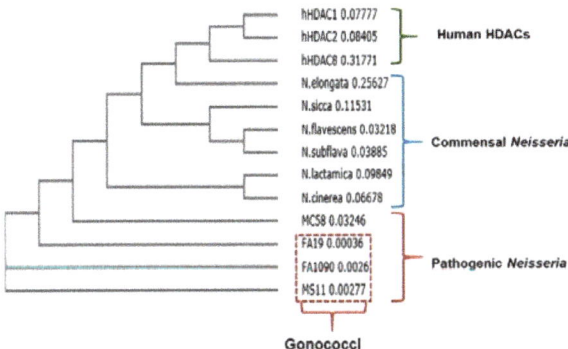

Figure 2. Evolution of *Neisseria gonorrhoeae* Gc-HDAC-like protein in human monocytes. Evolution of Neisseria Gc-HDAC-like protein compared to human HDACs. The multiple sequence alignment tool Clustal Omega was used to build the phylogenic tree (https://www.ebi.ac.uk/Tools/msa/clustalo/).

2.4. Expression of the Gonococcal HDAC-Encoding Gene

We examined whether the predicted *hdac* gene (GenBank: SCW18245.1; WP_050303785.1) could be expressed during growth in laboratory media and during infection of macrophages using qRT-PCR. The results showed that *hdac* is constitutively expressed at all growth phases (data not shown). To establish the biological significance of the predicted gene and whether it plays a role in pathogenesis, we examined its expression during infection of macrophages. Since Gc-HDAC has high 3D homology to human HDAC1 and peripheral monocytes express human HDAC1, we assessed the expression of both genes during infection of human peripheral monocytes. The results showed that the gonococcal *hdac* gene was expressed when monocytes from healthy donors were infected with live gonococcal strain FA19 at multiplicity of infection (MOI) of 10 (Figure 4). In contrast, gonococcal infection downregulated expression of the human HDAC1-encoding gene compared to uninfected monocytes (Figure 4). Therefore, we hypothesized that the Gc-HDAC-like protein may exert epigenetic modifications on host histones to suppress LL-37 gene expression or other determinants of innate immunity.

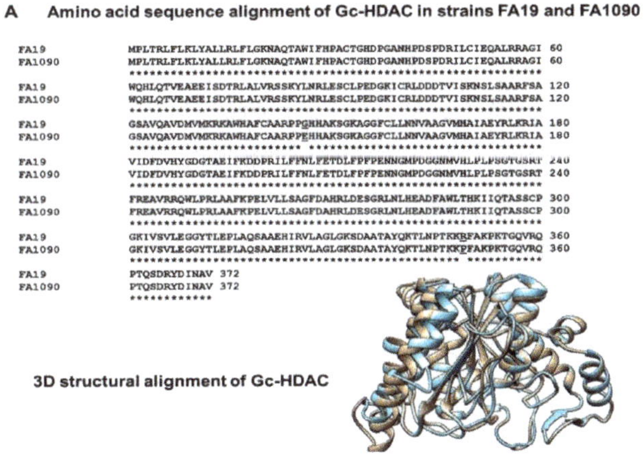

Figure 3. *Cont.*

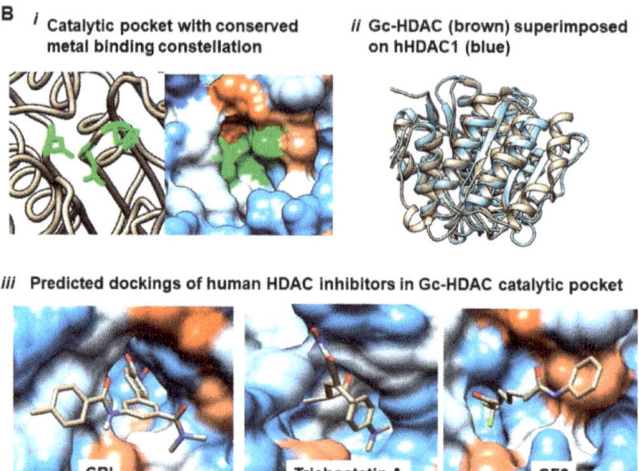

Figure 3. Computational analysis and in silico modeling of Gc-HDAC-like protein in *Neisseria gonorrhoeae*. (**A**): Amino acid sequence alignment of Gc-HDAC from gonococcal strains FA19 and FA1090 and their 3D structural alignment. (**B**): In silico modeling of Gc-HDAC-like protein: (i) predicted Gc-HDAC-like protein 3D structure revealing the catalytic pocket with the conserved metal binding constellation (green); (ii) predicted Gc-HDAC-like protein 3D structure (brown) is superimposed on human HDAC1 protein (blue) and (iii) predicted dockings of HDAC inhibitors CRI, trichostatin A and CF3 in Gc-HDAC catalytic pocket. Computational Gc-HDAC 3D protein structure and HDAC inhibitors dockings were predicted using I-TASSER, and PDB files were viewed using Chimera. The BS scores of top predictions for HDAC inhibitors CRI, TSA and CF3 are 1.51, 1.09 and 1.4, respectively. BS score definition by I-TASSER is a measure of local similarity (sequence and structure) between template binding site and predicted binding site in the query structure. Based on large-scale benchmarking analysis, a BS score >1 reflects a significant local match between the predicted and template binding site.

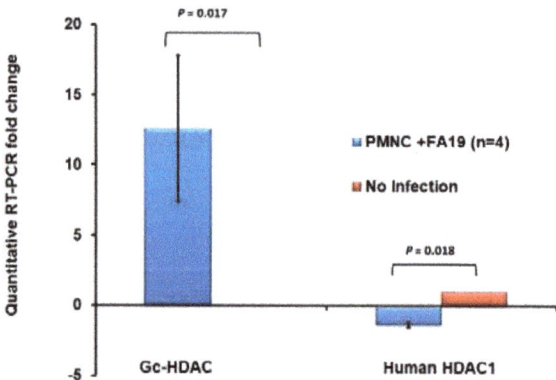

Figure 4. Expression of *Neisseria gonorrhoeae* Gc-HDAC-like protein during infection in peripheral human monocytes. Gc-HDAC gene expression during infection compared to human HDAC1 expression in peripheral human monocytes (PMNC) obtained from four healthy donors and infected with live gonococci at MOI 25 overnight. Gc-HDAC and hHDAC1 expression is assessed by quantitative RT-PCR normalized to β-actin gene expression and compared to noninfected PMNC (n = 4). p values were calculated using a Student's t-test in reference to noninfected PMNC.

To determine whether the production of Gc-HDAC-like protein impacts its intracellular survival ability, we performed macrophage bactericidal assays. For this purpose, we employed WT strain FA19 and a genetic derivative containing an insertionally inactivated *hdac* (*hdac::spc*). We first examined if loss of the *hdac* gene altered the growth characteristics of N. gonorrhoeae strain FA19. The overall data from in vitro cultures indicate that the Gc-HDAC-deficient mutant has a slight growth defect (data not shown). We examined if Gc-HDAC protein affects survival in macrophages. The results showed that the *hdac*-null mutant was slightly attenuated in murine RAW264 macrophages compared to the WT parent strain (Figure S1A). Similar results were observed in human THP-1 cells (data not shown). Furthermore, bacterial Gc-HDAC was found to be expressed during infection in human THP-1 macrophage-like cells (Figure S1B). In contrast, human HDAC1 was downregulated in infected THP-1 cells (Figure S1B), but this was independent of the Gc-HDAC. The downregulation of HDAC1 in THP-1 was similar to the observed data in peripheral human monocytes (Figure 4). Although the data suggest that Gc-HDAC-like protein may facilitate intracellular survival, it is possible that the moderate growth defect of the mutant is responsible for its reduced intracellular survival in macrophages.

2.5. N. Gonorrhoeae Exerts Epigenetic Modifications on Host Innate Immune Genes in Infected Macrophages

We hypothesized that the gonococcal HDAC-like protein could exert an epigenetic influence on host genes. Thus, potential acetylation of lysine could reduce histone binding to DNA and, therefore, allows transcription factors to bind to promoter elements, leading to gene regulation. In contrast, lysine deacetylation would lead to gene suppression. To examine whether gonococcal infection in macrophages causes epigenetic modifications, we performed a chromatin immune precipitation (ChIP) assay. Specifically, the alteration of histone 3 lysine 9 acetylation (H3K9ac) as a prominent epigenetic mark that changes during sepsis and infection in monocytes [23] was examined. We first examined the downregulation of human AMPs LL-37, HBD-1 and SLPI in THP-1 monocytes infected with live WT FA19, its isogenic Gc-HDAC-deficient and complemented strain. Using multiple MOIs (1, 5, 10, 25 and 50), we found that infection of target cells even at low MOI of 1 led to significant reduction in expression of AMP genes (Figure 5A). Importantly, reductions in gene expression show that AMPs were significantly downregulated in a Gc-HDAC-independent manner, although a slight but significant difference was observed when compared to parent strain FA19 (Figure 5A). This slight difference may be because the Gc-HDAC mutant has a moderate growth defect (see above). To examine the mechanism of CAMP gene downregulation, we then investigated epigenetic modifications at the promoters of host defense genes of LL-37 and HBD-1 during gonococcal infection with WT and the Gc-HDAC-deficient isogenic mutant. As expected, an H3K9ac epigenetic mark was not enriched at the promoters of host defense peptides LL-37 and HBD-1, suggesting gene silencing in a Gc-HDAC-independent manner (Figure 5B). Further, we investigated H3K9ac epigenetic mark enrichment in the promoters of other host innate immune genes involved in pathogen sensing and signaling; specifically, TLRs signaling pathways [24,25]. Results from the ChIP microarray showed that H3K9ac epigenetic mark is highly enriched in the promoters of proinflammatory and signaling genes of TLRs pathways in THP-1 cells infected with Gc-FA19 parent strain compared to its isogenic Gc-HDAC mutant or the noninfected THP-1 cells (Figure 6). Specifically, H3K9ac enrichment was observed in the promoters of the NFKB complex; other transcription factors like JNK, FOS and nuclear receptors; MAP kinases; TLRs and proinflammatory cytokines. H3K9ac epigenetic mark is highly enriched in the promoters of CD14, IL-10, type 1 IFN, TNFα and RELA 9p65 (Figure S2). Of note, the absence of Gc-HDAC differentially increased H3K9ac epigenetic mark enrichment in the promoters of IL-2, CCL2 (MCP-1), TLR1, SIGIRR, REL, MAPK8 and IKBKB. Most of these genes are negative regulators of the inflammatory response. Further, the observed epigenetic alterations at the promoters of host innate immune genes were confirmed by qRT-PCR using the TLR-focused RT2 microarray (Qiagen) to assess gene expression in infected macrophages (Figure S3). Taken together, the data suggest that Gc-HDAC-like protein in gonococci may contribute to histone modifications, consequently inducing proinflammatory genes while suppressing host defense peptides genes to facilitate survival and promote infection.

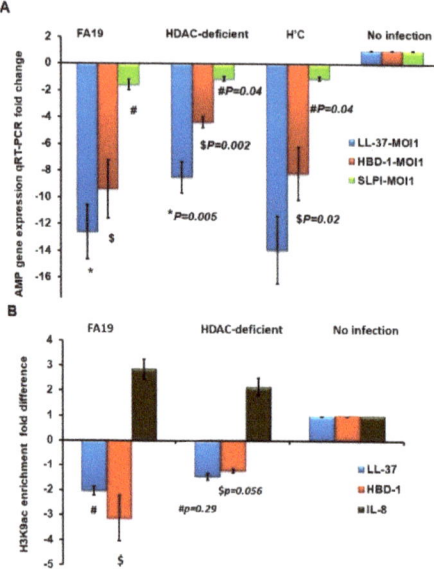

Figure 5. Expression of *Neisseria gonorrhoeae* AMPs gene expression in infected monocytes in the presence and absence of Gc-HDAC. (**A**): Expression of LL-37, HBD-1 and SLPI genes in THP-1 monocytes infected with WT strain FA19 or its isogenic Gc-HDAC-deficient mutant or the complemented H'C strain at MOI of 1 overnight (n = 3) was assessed using qRT-PCR. (**B**): H3K9ac epigenetic mark enrichment at the promoters of LL-37 and HBD-1 in THP-1 monocytes infected with WT strain FA19 or its isogenic Gc-HDAC-deficient mutant at MOI of 25 overnight (n = 3) was assessed using a ChIP assay. p values were calculated using a Student's t-test in reference to cells infected with the WT FA19 strain for LL-37 expression (*), HBD1 (#) and SLPI ($).

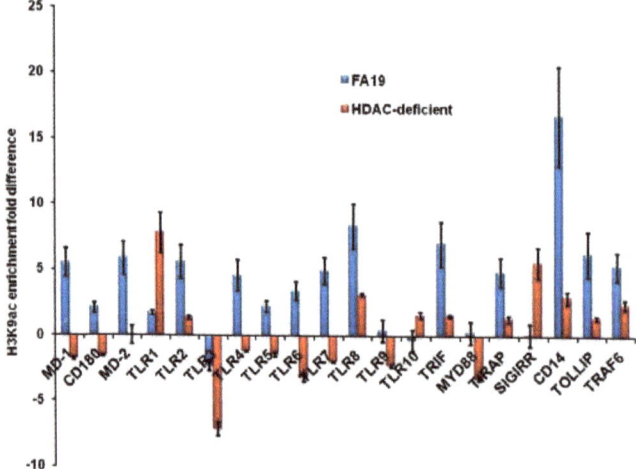

Figure 6. Gonococci exert epigenetic modifications in THP-1 monocytes. H3K9ac epigenetic mark enrichment at the promoters of genes involved in the TLRs signaling pathways. WT parent strain FA19: blue bars and isogenic HDAC-deficient mutant: red bars. Data are average of three independent ChIP experiments. p values were > 0.05 and were calculated using a Student's t-test comparing WT FA19 to the HDAC-deficient mutant.

3. Discussion

Epigenetic reprogramming in macrophages is termed trained innate immunity, and it regulates immune tolerance and limits tissue damage during infection [26–29]. However, maladaptive states of trained immunity cause sepsis and hyper-inflammation. *N. gonorrhoeae* is known to evade multiple host defense systems to facilitate survival and promote infection. Here, we show that gonococcal infection of human macrophages led to significant reduction in host defense CAMP genes expression encoding LL-37, HBD-1 and SLPI. We also show for the first time that *N. gonorrhoeae* infection in macrophages can induce epigenetic modifications on host chromatin through a Gc-HDAC-independent process. Our data suggest that gonococcal infection in macrophages exerts epigenetic modifications to modify host gene expression. The maladaptive state of trained immunity impacts clearance of pathogens, as well as the development of optimal adaptive immune responses. Gonococcal infections are asymptomatic in 50%–70% of cases among females, as well as in some cases of male rectal gonorrhea [30,31]. However, gonococcal infections associate with severe pelvic inflammatory disease and infertility, in addition to increasing the risk of HIV transmission and other sexually transmitted infections like chlamydia [31]. Our data showed that gonococcal *hdac* is constitutively expressed at all growth phases. Interestingly, a recent study analyzed the complete gonococcal transcriptome response during anaerobic growth of gonococci and reported that an ORF identical to *hdac* was upregulated more than 4-fold compared to aerobic growth conditions [32]. This upregulation of gene expression under anaerobic conditions is physiologically relevant to gonococcal infections in fallopian tubes and upper genital tract causing pelvic inflammatory disease, which is a severe and symptomatic infection. Therefore, the Gc-HDAC-like protein may play a role in promoting ascending gonococcal infections. Further, gonococcal infections do not confer protective immunity following natural infections [33]. Therefore, we postulate that gonococcal infections induce a maladaptive state of trained immunity in the human host.

The exact molecular mechanisms by which gonococci exert epigenetic modifications are not clear. *N. gonorrhoeae* does not possess SET-containing domain effectors that are known to exert epigenetic modifications on host chromatin [34,35]. Using the bioinformatics approach, we identified a gene that encodes a histone deacetylase-like enzyme (Gc-HDAC) that shares high 3D homology to human HDAC1, HDAC2 and HDAC8. In eukaryotic cells, HDACs suppress gene expression by condensing chromatin packing consequently, preventing transcription factors from binding to gene promoters [21]. We tested our hypothesis, that the Gc-HDAC protein exerts epigenetic modifications on host histones to suppress LL-37 gene expression, which facilitates immune evasion and promotes intracellular survival. Of note, gonococcal infection in macrophages downregulated the expression of human HDAC1, the most commonly expressed human HDAC in myeloid cells [36–39], suggesting epigenetic modulation (Figure 4 and Figure S1B). This observation is novel and consistent with the notion that *N. gonorrhoeae* can modulate host responses for the purpose of immune evasion [16]. Although the Gc-HDAC mutant is attenuated, we concluded that the observed epigenetic modifications are Gc-HDAC-independent. Therefore, the exact molecular mechanism underlying these epigenetic modifications remains unclear. Bioinformatics analyses is ongoing to identify other potential effectors that *N. gonorrhoeae* may harbor that are directly causing these epigenetic modifications. Further, expanded epigenetic modifications profiling beyond epigenetic mark H3K9ac to investigate other epigenetic marks, such as H4K16 acetylation and H3K9 trimethylation [40], may shed a light on the possible role of Gc-HDAC in modifying host chromatin and promoting the gonococcal modulation of and evasion of host responses.

4. Materials and Methods

Reagents: RPMI 1640 medium, Dulbecco's modified Eagle's medium (D-MEM), fetal bovine serum (FBS), penicillin/streptomycin, sodium pyruvate and nonessential amino acids were obtained from Cellgro Mediatech (Herdon, VA). Chromatin immune precipitation ChIP reagents EpiTect® ChIP kit and ChIP antibodies were purchased from Qiagen (Hilden, Germany). HDAC inhibitors trichostatin

A and sodium butyrate TSA were purchased from Sigma (St Louis, MO, USA). Other HDAC inhibitors valproic acid and entinostat were kind gifts from Dr. Seth Brodie (Winship Cancer Center, Emory University School of Medicine, Atlanta, GA, USA).

Computational analysis: A bioinformatics blast search for conserved SET or HDAC domains was performed on all available *Neisseria spp.*-sequenced genomes using the "Delta Blast" search function available by the National Center for Biotechnology Information, known as NCBI (https://blast.ncbi.nlm.nih.gov/Blast.cgi?PROGRAM=blastp&PAGE_TYPE=BlastSearch&BLAST_PROGRAMS=deltaBlast&RESET_PROGRAM=on&RID=W4K9E36F014). We employed computational modeling to predict the GC-HDAC-like protein structure-function. The amino acid sequence of the identified GC-HDAC-like protein sequence of 372 amino acids was deposited into two different molecular modeling softwares, I-TASSER [41] and Phyre Protein Fold [42], to predict protein 3D structure. The predicted protein databank (PDB) files were then visualized using Chimera software [43]. Computational analysis was performed on GC-HDAC from gonococcal strains FA19, FA1090, MS11 and GD12.

The following HDAC inhibitors were predicted to dock in the Gc-HDAC enzyme catalytic pocket: CF3: 9,9,9-TRIFLUORO-8-OXO-N-PHENYLNONANAMIDE; CRI: 5-(4-METHYL-BENZOYLAMINO)-BIPHENYL-3,4′-DICARBOXYLIC ACID 3-DIMETHYLAMIDE-4′-HYDROXYAMIDE and TSA: trichostatin A. HDAC inhibitors compound structures are available at https://pubchem.ncbi.nlm.nih.gov/compound.

Construction of genetic derivatives: The *hdac* gene was amplified using primers 0187pac1 (5′-GATCTTAATTAATATGCCGTCTGCACCCCC-3′) and 0187pme1 (5′-GATCGTTTAAACGAAAACCGAATCGGCTTCAG -3′) and FA19 genomic DNA as the template. The corresponding 1118 bp PCR product and the pGCC4 vector [44] were digested by Pac1 and Pme1 and then ligated overnight at 16 °C. The ligation was then transformed into *Escherichia coli* DH5α. Transformants were verified by PCR, and a verified transformant was selected for further study. After growth overnight, DNA from the transformant was extracted using a Qiaprep column, as described by the manufacturer (Qiagen), and its insert was sequenced. pGCC4 *hdac* was digested by Xho1, and a spectinomycin (Spc) cassette was inserted in the Xho1 site. The ligation was transformed into *E. coli* DH5α, and transformants were selected on GC plates supplemented with 60 μg/mL of Spc and verified by PCR. After growth overnight, pGCC4*hdac::spc* was extracted using a Qiaprep column, as described by the manufacturer (Qiagen). A PCR was performed using primers 0187pac1 and 0187pme1 and pGCC4*hdac::spc* as the template. This 3118 bp PCR product was then transformed into FA19, as previously described [45]; transformants were selected on GC plates supplemented with 60 μg/mL of Spc. FA19*hdac::spc* transformants were verified by PCR. One clone was selected and transformed by pGCC4*hdac*; transformants were selected on GC plates supplemented with 1 μg/mL of erythromycin (ery). One FA19*hdac::SpcC′* clone was selected, and the insertion of the wild-type copy of *hdac* at the *lctP/aspC* locus was verified by PCR and sequencing.

Construction of FA19Str^R*hdac::Spec* and FA19Str^R*hdac::SpcC′*: DNA from strain FA19Str^R [46] was extracted [47] and transformed into FA19*hdac::spc* and FA19*hdac::SpcC′*, as previously described [45]. Transformants were selected on GC plates supplemented with 1600 μg/mL of streptomycin. Four transformants from each transformation were selected, and the *rpsL* gene was PCR-amplified using primers rpsLF (5′-CGTTATGCTTGACTGTCTGC-3′) and rpsLR (5′-TCTATTCCCATGAATACCCAAT-3′) and sequenced.

Bacterial growth curves: To investigate whether the deletion of HDAC gene impacts bacterial growth, the growth rate of the parent strain FA19 to the HDAC-deficient isogenic and complemented mutants were compared, as previously described [24]. Briefly, WT strain FA19 (wild-type; WT), its isogenic mutant *hdac::spc* strain and complemented strain (HDAC-C′) strains were grown as pilus-positive, opacity-negative colony variants on GC agar containing defined Supplements I and II and 1 mM isopropyl β-D-1-thiogalactopyranoside (IPTG) under 5.0% (v/v) CO_2 at 37 °C, as described by Shafer et al. [45]. Gonococci were grown in GC broth with supplements and 0.043% (w/v) sodium bicarbonate at 37 °C in a shaking water bath. The viability of Gc cultures was determined using dilution plating onto GC agar, and colony forming units (CFU) were enumerated after 24 h of incubation at 37 °C in a CO_2 incubator. Gc grown on agar plates were resuspended in GC broth and harvested by centrifugation at 5000× g for 10 min. The bacterial pellet was washed twice with PBS and resuspended in 10 mL of D-MEM tissue culture medium without antibiotics to prepare a live Gc inoculum for macrophage infection experiments (see below) [7].

Cell cultures: THP-1 human macrophage-like monocytic cells were obtained from the American Type Culture Collection (ATCC, Manassas, VA) and grown in RPMI 1640 with L-glutamate supplemented with 10% (v/v) FBS, 50 IU/mL of penicillin and 50 µg/mL of streptomycin. Culture flasks were incubated at 37 °C with humidity and 5% (v/v) CO_2. Murine macrophages (RAW264 from ATCC) were grown in D-MEM supplemented and incubated as noted above.

Macrophage infection assay: Freshly grown human THP-1 macrophage-like monocytic cells (in the absence of antibiotics) were adjusted to one million cells/mL, then transferred into 8-well tissue culture plates (2 mL/well) and infected with live Gc FA19, Gc-*hdac*::*spc* or its complemented strain at multiplicity of infection (MOI) of 25, 10, 5 and 1, then incubated overnight at 37 °C with 5% (v/v) CO_2. Uninfected cells in triplicate wells were also incubated simultaneously and were used as a minus infection control. Supernatants from infected or uninfected macrophages were harvested and saved at −20 °C for determination of chemokines release, and cells were washed with PBS, pelleted (1000× g for 5 min) and saved at −80 °C for Western blot analysis.

Isolation of peripheral monocytes: We previously published the detailed protocol of isolating peripheral monocytes from healthy donors in our previous paper [7]. The study was deemed exempt from the Institutional Review Board (IRB) at Emory University since peripheral monocytes were completely de-identified without any link to donors' identification. Briefly, whole blood (15 mL with EDTA) was collected from healthy donors after obtaining written informed consent under Emory University IRB approval to collect healthy donors' plasma for other unrelated studies. Peripheral monocytes were isolated using Ficoll-density gradient centrifugation (Histopaque 1077, Sigma-Aldrich, St Louis, MO, USA), as described [7]. Primary peripheral monocytes were infected with live GC-FA19 at an MOI of 10 and incubated overnight. Monocytes were harvested for RNA isolation, and gene expression was measured by quantitative RT-PCR.

Macrophage bactericidal assay: To determine whether the Gc-HDAC protein plays a role in the survival of Gc in association with macrophages, we employed murine RAW264 macrophage bactericidal assays, as previously described [7,9]. Briefly, freshly grown Gc strains were adjusted to an OD600 of 1.0 (~1 × 10^8 CFU/mL) in antibiotic-free D-MEM medium containing 10% heat-inactivated fetal bovine serum (FBS). Macrophages were also freshly grown, washed and adjusted to 1 million cells/mL in antibiotic-free D-MEM medium containing 10% FBS. Since these RAW264 macrophages are adherent, cells were seeded in 24-well tissue culture plates (1 million cells/well) and allowed to adhere overnight prior to infection with live gonococci at an MOI of 25, as described above. After one hour of initiated phagocytosis at 37 °C, adherent RAW264 cells were washed three times with antibiotic-free medium containing 10% heat-inactivated FBS, and all fluids were carefully removed without disturbing the adherent macrophages. One ml of fresh antibiotic-free medium containing 10% heat-inactivated FBS was added to each well, and infected cells were further incubated for 1 h. Extracellular Gc were removed by washing adherent macrophages three times with D-MEM medium. Viable intracellular (or tightly adherent) Gc were assessed by serial plating of macrophage cultures lysed using 0.01% triton X-100 in PBS, as previously described [7].

ChIP assay: To investigate whether *N. gonorrhoeae* exerts epigenetic modifications on host histones, a chromatin immune precipitation (ChIP) assay was performed. Briefly, histone modification patterns in the 1000 bp proximal promoter regions of LL-37 and HBD-1 genes were analyzed by ChIP and qPCR [48]. THP-1 cells were infected with gonococci at an MOI of 25, as described above. All cells were incubated for 16 h and cross-linked with 1% formaldehyde. THP-1 cells were lysed with lysing buffer (50 mM Tris–HCl, pH 8.0, 10 mM EDTA, 1% (wt/vol) SDS, protease inhibitor cocktail (1:100 dilution from 100× stock, Thermo Scientific, Hanover Park, IL, USA), 1 mM 189 PMSF, 20 mM Na-butyrate), and nuclei was harvested by centrifugation at 4000× *g* for 5 min at 4 °C. Chromatin was sheared on ice with a Microson Ultrasonic Cell Disruptor, XL (Heat System, Newtown, CT, USA). Specific histone modifications antibodies: anti-acetyl-Histone H3 (Lys9) (Cat# 07-352), anti-trimethyl-Histone H3 (Lys9) (Cat# 07-442) or anti-trimethyl-Histone H3 (Lys4) (Cat# 07-473) (all from Millipore, Hayward, CA, USA) conjugated to protein A /G Dynabeads (Life Technologies, Carlsbad, CA, USA) were used to pull down modified histone bound to DNA. These specific antibodies were incubated with sheared chromatin at 4 °C for 2 h. Isotype-matched antibody was included as negative ChIP control. The precipitated histone DNA was subjected to proteinase K digestion (50 µg/mL) for 30 min at 56 °C. DNA was purified using Qiaquick nucleotide removal columns from Qiagen (Hilden, Germany). The harvested DNA was quantified by qPCR using primers specific for the LL-37 (*camp*) and HBD-1 (*hbd-1*) gene promoter regions. The following primers were used in ChIP PCR quantitation: c-LL-37-F: 5'-GGCTTGGGAACATTTTGAGA-3' and c-LL-37-R: 5'-ATCCCCTTCTGCATCCTTCT-3' and c-HBD-1-F: 5'-TCCAGAAACCCCATCAGAAC-3' and c-HBD-1-R: 5'-CCGCTGGATTTAGCTTTCAG-3'. The relative fold change of DNA was calculated by comparing the percentage of precipitated DNA (% input) in infected THP-1 cells to that in the uninfected control cells. Antibodies used in the ChIP assay are specific to histone modifications, such as acetylated and trimethylated lysine residues in histone tails.

Host Cell gene expression using TLR-focused microarray (RT^2 Real-Time PCR array): One million cell/mL THP-1 cells were transferred to 12-well formats and then infected with *N. gonorrhoeae* strain FA19 or its Gc-HDAC isogenic mutant at MOI of 1, 10 and 15. Uninfected cells were used as controls for basal gene expression level. Cells were further incubated overnight at 37 °C under 5% CO_2. RNA was isolated using RNeasy Mini kits (Qiagen, Hilden, Germany), as previously described [49]. Briefly, cells were harvested in RLT buffer, passed over QiaShredder columns, and the resulting lysate was mixed in 70% ethanol, then was passed over RNeasy columns (Qiagen). Isolated RNA was then reverse-transcribed to cDNA using a First Strand kit from Qiagen. The generated cDNA was diluted with 91 µL of ddH_2O to each 20 µL of cDNA synthesis reaction. The experimental cocktail for real-time PCR was prepared in a sterile boat as follows: 1275 µL of 2X SYBR Green PCR Master Mix (Applied Biosystems, Foster City, CA, USA), 102 µL of diluted cDNA and 1173 µL of ddH_2O. Real-time PCR was then performed using RT^2 Profiler^{TM} PCR Array (Qiagen) in 96-well format pre-loaded with the primers. Human Toll-like receptor signaling pathway and human apoptosis pathway RT^2 Profiler^{TM} PCR Arrays profile the expression of 84 genes related to the TLR-mediated signal transduction pathway. In addition to primers, the array contains all positive and negative controls required for the real-time PCR procedure. To start the real-time PCR reaction, 25 µL of experimental cocktail mix was carefully added to each well in the RT^2 PCR Array using a multichannel pipette, then was tightly sealed with the optical adhesive film. The PCR parameters were set as follows: 2 min at 50 °C, 10 min at 95 °C and 45 cycles of 95 °C for 15 s, followed by 1 min at 62 °C. For data analysis, the Excel-based PCR Array data analysis template (downloaded from this link: https://www.qiagen.com was used. Gene expression profiles were automatically calculated from threshold cycle data generated from the real-time instrument, and any C_t value equal or greater than 35 was considered negative.

Quantitative RT-PCR analysis: RNA was extracted from infected and uninfected macrophages using an RNeasy kit and was transcribed to cDNA using a reverse transcriptase kit from Qiagen, as previously described [7]. The relative gene expression was normalized to uninfected controls, and primers used in qRT-PCR were previously described [7]. For this study the following primers used in qRT-PCR were: LL-37-F: GGGCACACTGTCTCCTTCAC and LL-37-R: TCGGATGCTA**A**CCTCTACCG. The following primer sets (Quantitect® Primer Assay) were purchased from Qiagen: human HBD-1 (Hs_DEFB_1_SG), human SLPI (Hs_SLPI_1_SG), human HBD-5 (Hs_DEFB105A_3_SG) and hHDAC1 (Hs_HDAC1_1_SG).

Cytokine and Chemokine release quantification: In order to determine whether the production of Gc-HDAC impacted the magnitude of the innate immune response, cytokines and chemokines released from infected macrophages were quantified. Briefly, freshly grown human THP-1 monocytic cells were harvested and adjusted to one million cells/mL without antibiotics, transferred into 6-well tissue culture plates (3 mL/well) and infected with viable strains FA19, Gc-HDAC::spc and the complemented strain Gc-HDAC'C at a multiplicity of infection (MOI) of 1, 5, 10 and 25. Cells were then incubated at 37 °C with 5% CO_2 for 5 h or overnight. Uninfected cells in triplicate wells were also incubated simultaneously and used as a no-infection control. Supernatants were harvested and saved at −20 °C for determination of cytokine release, and cells were collected for RNA extraction. Cytokine/chemokine releases in the supernatants collected from infected macrophages were assessed using the multiplex ELISA panel from Invivogen (San Diego, CA, USA), and the following cytokines: TNFα, IL-1β, IL-6, IL-4, IL-12p70, IL-17, IL-10, IFNγ and IFNα and chemokines: IL-8, IP-10, MCP-1, RANTES, Eotaxin, MIP1α and MIP1β were included. Briefly, 50 μL of supernatants were mixed with the multiplex magnetic beads precoated with cytokines and chemokines-specific antibodies in buffer, and ELISA was performed using the Luminex array.

In vitro fitness analysis of gonococci: Broth cultures (25 mL GC broth (GCB) supplemented with Kellogg's supplements I and II and 5 mM $NaHCO_3$) of wild-type [29] parent FA19 or Gc-HDAC-deficient mutant strains (passaged once) were prepared at an OD_{600} of 0.05. A third broth culture with an equal mixture of both parent and mutant strains (i.e., competitive culture) was also prepared with the same starting OD_{600}. Over an 8-h period, optical density of the cultures was measured every hour, while bacterial counts were assessed every 2 h using plate dilution. For the latter, plates were incubated at 37 °C with 7% CO_2 for 48 h before counting CFUs. The competitive index was calculated using the following equation: output ratio divided by input ratio, where the output ratio is the number of mutant CFU divided by those from the WT parent CFU at a particular time point, while the input ratio is the number of mutant CFU divided by the WT parent CFU in the inoculum (T = 0) of the competitive culture.

Statistical analysis: Mean values ± SD (standard deviation) and p values (Student's t-test) of at least three independent determinations were calculated with Microsoft Excel software.

Supplementary Materials: The following are available online at http://www.mdpi.com/2076-0817/9/2/132/s1: Figure S1: Survival of gonococcal strain FA19 and its isogenic Gc-HDAC deficient mutant in macrophages. Figure S2: Gonococci exert epigenetic modifications in THP-1 monocytes. Figure S3: Pro-inflammatory genes expression is highly upregulated in macrophages infected with live gonococci.

Author Contributions: Conceptualization, S.M.Z.; methodology, S.M.Z. and C.E.R.-L.; software, S.M.Z.; validation, S.M.Z. and C.E.R.-L.; formal analysis, S.M.Z., C.E.R.-L. and W.M.S.; investigation, S.M.Z., C.E.R.-L. and W.M.S.; resources, X.X.; data curation, S.M.Z., C.E.R.-L. and W.M.S.; writing—original draft preparation, S.M.Z.; writing—review and editing, S.M.Z., C.E.R.-L. and W.M.S.; project administration, S.M.Z. and W.M.S. and funding acquisition, S.M.Z. and W.M.S. All authors have read and agreed to the published version of the manuscript.

Funding: This research was funded by a Development Research Program grant to S.M.Z. from the Henry M. Jackson Foundation through an NIH grant 1U19AI113170-01 (Ann E. Jerse, PI, Uniformed Services University, Bethesda, MD, USA) and a VA Merit Award grant (510 1BX000112-07) to W.M.S. from the Biomedical Laboratory Research and Development Service of the Department of Veterans Affairs. W.M.S. was supported by a Senior Research Career Award from the Biomedical Laboratory Research and Development Service of the Department of Veterans Affairs. The content of this article is solely the responsibility of the authors and does not necessarily represent the official views of the National Institutes of Health or the Department of Veterans Affairs or the United States Government.

Acknowledgments: The authors thank Ann E. Jerse, Uniformed Services University, Bethesda, MD for critically discussing and reviewing the manuscript.

Conflicts of Interest: The authors declare no conflict of interest. The funders had no role in the design of the study; in the collection, analyses, or interpretation of data; in the writing of the manuscript; or in the decision to publish the results.

References

1. Rowley, J.; Vander Hoorn, S.; Korenromp, E.; Low, N.; Unemo, M.; Abu-Raddad, L.J.; Chico, R.M.; Smolak, A.; Newman, L.; Gottlieb, S.; et al. Chlamydia, gonorrhoea, trichomoniasis and syphilis: Global prevalence and incidence estimates, 2016. *Bull. World Health Organ.* **2019**, *97*, 548–562. [CrossRef]

2. CDC. Trends in aging—United States and worldwide. *MMWR Morb. Mortal. Wkly. Rep.* **2003**, *52*, 101–104.
3. Tapsall, J.W.; Shultz, T.; Limnios, E.; Munro, R.; Mercer, J.; Porritt, R.; Griffith, J.; Hogg, G.; Lum, G.; Lawrence, A.; et al. Surveillance of antibiotic resistance in invasive isolates of Neisseria meningitidis in Australia 1994–1999. *Pathology* **2001**, *33*, 359–361. [CrossRef] [PubMed]
4. Shultz, T.R.; Tapsall, J.W.; White, P.A. Correlation of in vitro susceptibilities to newer quinolones of naturally occurring quinolone-resistant Neisseria gonorrhoeae strains with changes in GyrA and ParC. *Antimicrob. Agents Chemother.* **2001**, *45*, 734–738. [CrossRef] [PubMed]
5. WHO. *Emergence of Multi-Drug Resistant Neisseria Gonorrhoeae—Threat of Global Rise in Untreated Sexually Transmitted Infections*; WHO: Geneva, Switzerland, 2011.
6. WHO. *Global Priority List of Antibiotic-Resistant Bacteria to Guide Research, Discovery, and Development of New Antibiotics*; WHO: Geneva, Switzerland, 2017.
7. Zughaier, S.M.; Kandler, J.L.; Shafer, W.M. Neisseria gonorrhoeae modulates iron-limiting innate immune defenses in macrophages. *PLoS ONE* **2014**, *9*, e87688. [CrossRef] [PubMed]
8. Criss, A.K.; Seifert, H.S. A bacterial siren song: Intimate interactions between Neisseria and neutrophils. *Nat. Rev. Microbiol.* **2012**, *10*, 178–190. [CrossRef] [PubMed]
9. Zughaier, S.M.; Kandler, J.L.; Balthazar, J.T.; Shafer, W.M. Phosphoethanolamine modification of neisseria gonorrhoeae lipid A reduces autophagy flux in macrophages. *PLoS ONE* **2015**, *10*, e0144347. [CrossRef] [PubMed]
10. Kandler, J.L.; Joseph, S.J.; Balthazar, J.T.; Dhulipala, V.; Read, T.D.; Jerse, A.E.; Shafer, W.M. Phase-variable expression of lptA modulates the resistance of Neisseria gonorrhoeae to cationic antimicrobial peptides. *Antimicrob. Agents Chemother.* **2014**, *58*, 4230–4233. [CrossRef]
11. Abu El-Asrar, A.M.; Struyf, S.; Descamps, F.J.; Al-Obeidan, S.A.; Proost, P.; Van Damme, J.; Opdenakker, G.; Geboes, K. Chemokines and gelatinases in the aqueous humor of patients with active uveitis. *Am. J. Ophthalmol.* **2004**, *138*, 401–411. [CrossRef]
12. Lewis, L.A.; Shafer, W.M.; Dutta Ray, T.; Ram, S.; Rice, P.A. Phosphoethanolamine residues on the lipid A moiety of Neisseria gonorrhoeae lipooligosaccharide modulate binding of complement inhibitors and resistance to complement killing. *Infect. Immun.* **2013**, *81*, 33–42. [CrossRef]
13. Handing, J.W.; Criss, A.K. The lipooligosaccharide-modifying enzyme LptA enhances gonococcal defence against human neutrophils. *Cell. Microbiol.* **2015**, *17*, 910–921. [CrossRef] [PubMed]
14. Packiam, M.; Yedery, R.D.; Begum, A.A.; Carlson, R.W.; Ganguly, J.; Sempowski, G.D.; Ventevogel, M.S.; Shafer, W.M.; Jerse, A.E. Phosphoethanolamine decoration of Neisseria gonorrhoeae lipid A plays a dual immunostimulatory and protective role during experimental genital tract infection. *Infect. Immun.* **2014**, *82*, 2170–2179. [CrossRef] [PubMed]
15. Hobbs, M.M.; Anderson, J.E.; Balthazar, J.T.; Kandler, J.L.; Carlson, R.W.; Ganguly, J.; Begum, A.A.; Duncan, J.A.; Lin, J.T.; Sparling, P.F.; et al. Lipid A's structure mediates neisseria gonorrhoeae fitness during experimental infection of mice and men. *mBio* **2013**, *4*. [CrossRef] [PubMed]
16. Bergman, P.; Johansson, L.; Asp, V.; Plant, L.; Gudmundsson, G.H.; Jonsson, A.B.; Agerberth, B. Neisseria gonorrhoeae downregulates expression of the human antimicrobial peptide LL-37. *Cell. Microbiol.* **2005**, *7*, 1009–1017. [CrossRef]
17. Strahl, B.D.; Allis, C.D. The language of covalent histone modifications. *Nature* **2000**, *403*, 41–45. [CrossRef]
18. Duan, Q.; Chen, H.; Costa, M.; Dai, W. Phosphorylation of H3S10 blocks the access of H3K9 by specific antibodies and histone methyltransferase. Implication in regulating chromatin dynamics and epigenetic inheritance during mitosis. *J. Biol. Chem.* **2008**, *283*, 33585–33590. [CrossRef]
19. Liu, H.; Duan, Y. Effects of posttranslational modifications on the structure and dynamics of histone H3 N-terminal peptide. *Biophys. J.* **2008**, *94*, 4579–4585. [CrossRef]
20. Finnin, M.S.; Donigian, J.R.; Cohen, A.; Richon, V.M.; Rifkind, R.A.; Marks, P.A.; Breslow, R.; Pavletich, N.P. Structures of a histone deacetylase homologue bound to the TSA and SAHA inhibitors. *Nature* **1999**, *401*, 188–193. [CrossRef]
21. Moser, M.A.; Hagelkruys, A.; Seiser, C. Transcription and beyond: The role of mammalian class I lysine deacetylases. *Chromosoma* **2014**, *123*, 67–78. [CrossRef]
22. Hildmann, C.; Ninkovic, M.; Dietrich, R.; Wegener, D.; Riester, D.; Zimmermann, T.; Birch, O.M.; Bernegger, C.; Loidl, P.; Schwienhorst, A. A new amidohydrolase from Bordetella or Alcaligenes strain FB188 with similarities to histone deacetylases. *J. Bacteriol.* **2004**, *186*, 2328–2339. [CrossRef]

23. Iglesias, M.J.; Reilly, S.J.; Emanuelsson, O.; Sennblad, B.; Pirmoradian Najafabadi, M.; Folkersen, L.; Malarstig, A.; Lagergren, J.; Eriksson, P.; Hamsten, A.; et al. Combined chromatin and expression analysis reveals specific regulatory mechanisms within cytokine genes in the macrophage early immune response. *PLoS ONE* **2012**, *7*, e32306.
24. Kumar, H.; Kawai, T.; Akira, S. Toll-like receptors and innate immunity. *Biochem. Biophys. Res. Commun.* **2009**, *388*, 621–625. [CrossRef] [PubMed]
25. Kawai, T.; Akira, S. The roles of TLRs, RLRs and NLRs in pathogen recognition. *Int. Immunol.* **2009**, *21*, 317–337. [CrossRef]
26. van der Meer, J.W.; Joosten, L.A.; Riksen, N.; Netea, M.G. Trained immunity: A smart way to enhance innate immune defence. *Mol. Immunol.* **2015**, *68*, 40–44. [CrossRef] [PubMed]
27. Blok, B.A.; Arts, R.J.; van Crevel, R.; Benn, C.S.; Netea, M.G. Trained innate immunity as underlying mechanism for the long-term, nonspecific effects of vaccines. *J. Leukoc. Biol.* **2015**, *98*, 347–356. [CrossRef]
28. Ifrim, D.C.; Quintin, J.; Meerstein-Kessel, L.; Plantinga, T.S.; Joosten, L.A.; van der Meer, J.W.; van de Veerdonk, F.L.; Netea, M.G. Defective trained immunity in patients with STAT-1-dependent chronic mucocutaneaous candidiasis. *Clin. Exp. Immunol.* **2015**, *181*, 434–440. [CrossRef]
29. Kleinnijenhuis, J.; van Crevel, R.; Netea, M.G. Trained immunity: Consequences for the heterologous effects of BCG vaccination. *Trans. R. Soc. Trop. Med. Hyg.* **2015**, *109*, 29–35. [CrossRef]
30. Walker, C.K.; Sweet, R.L. Gonorrhea infection in women: Prevalence, effects, screening, and management. *Int. J. Women's Health* **2011**, *3*, 197–206.
31. Vodstrcil, L.A.; Fairley, C.K.; Fehler, G.; Leslie, D.; Walker, J.; Bradshaw, C.S.; Hocking, J.S. Trends in chlamydia and gonorrhea positivity among heterosexual men and men who have sex with men attending a large urban sexual health service in Australia, 2002–2009. *BMC Infect. Dis.* **2011**, *11*, 158. [CrossRef]
32. Isabella, V.M.; Clark, V.L. Deep sequencing-based analysis of the anaerobic stimulon in Neisseria gonorrhoeae. *BMC Genom.* **2011**, *12*, 51. [CrossRef]
33. Jerse, A.E.; Bash, M.C.; Russell, M.W. Vaccines against gonorrhea: Current status and future challenges. *Vaccine* **2014**, *32*, 1579–1587. [CrossRef] [PubMed]
34. Rolando, M.; Sanulli, S.; Rusniok, C.; Gomez-Valero, L.; Bertholet, C.; Sahr, T.; Margueron, R.; Buchrieser, C. Legionella pneumophila effector RomA uniquely modifies host chromatin to repress gene expression and promote intracellular bacterial replication. *Cell Host Microbe* **2013**, *13*, 395–405. [CrossRef] [PubMed]
35. Crotty Alexander, L.E.; Marsh, B.J.; Timmer, A.M.; Lin, A.E.; Zainabadi, K.; Czopik, A.; Guarente, L.; Nizet, V. Myeloid cell sirtuin-1 expression does not alter host immune responses to Gram-negative endotoxemia or Gram-positive bacterial infection. *PLoS ONE* **2013**, *8*, e84481. [CrossRef] [PubMed]
36. Borutinskaite, V.; Navakauskiene, R. The histone deacetylase inhibitor BML-210 influences gene and protein expression in human promyelocytic leukemia NB4 cells via epigenetic reprogramming. *Int. J. Mol. Sci.* **2015**, *16*, 18252–18269. [CrossRef] [PubMed]
37. Kallsen, K.; Andresen, E.; Heine, H. Histone deacetylase (HDAC) 1 controls the expression of beta defensin 1 in human lung epithelial cells. *PLoS ONE* **2012**, *7*, e50000. [CrossRef] [PubMed]
38. Garcia-Garcia, J.C.; Barat, N.C.; Trembley, S.J.; Dumler, J.S. Epigenetic silencing of host cell defense genes enhances intracellular survival of the rickettsial pathogen Anaplasma phagocytophilum. *PLoS Pathog.* **2009**, *5*, e1000488. [CrossRef]
39. Garcia-Garcia, J.C.; Rennoll-Bankert, K.E.; Pelly, S.; Milstone, A.M.; Dumler, J.S. Silencing of host cell CYBB gene expression by the nuclear effector AnkA of the intracellular pathogen Anaplasma phagocytophilum. *Infect. Immun.* **2009**, *77*, 2385–2391. [CrossRef]
40. Bierne, H.; Hamon, M.; Cossart, P. Epigenetics and bacterial infections. *Cold Spring Harb. Perspect. Med.* **2012**, *2*, a010272. [CrossRef]
41. Zhang, Y. I-TASSER server for protein 3D structure prediction. *BMC Bioinform.* **2008**, *9*, 40. [CrossRef]
42. Kelley, L.A.; Sternberg, M.J. Protein structure prediction on the Web: A case study using the phyre server. *Nat. Protoc.* **2009**, *4*, 363–371. [CrossRef]
43. Pettersen, E.F.; Goddard, T.D.; Huang, C.C.; Couch, G.S.; Greenblatt, D.M.; Meng, E.C.; Ferrin, T.E. UCSF Chimera—A visualization system for exploratory research and analysis. *J. Comput. Chem.* **2004**, *25*, 1605–1612. [CrossRef] [PubMed]

44. Skaar, E.P.; Lecuyer, B.; Lenich, A.G.; Lazio, M.P.; Perkins-Balding, D.; Seifert, H.S.; Karls, A.C. Analysis of the piv recombinase-related gene family of Neisseria gonorrhoeae. *J. Bacteriol.* **2005**, *187*, 1276–1286. [CrossRef] [PubMed]
45. Shafer, W.M.; Joiner, K.; Guymon, L.F.; Cohen, M.S.; Sparling, P.F. Serum sensitivity of Neisseria gonorrhoeae: The role of lipopolysaccharide. *J. Infect. Dis.* **1984**, *149*, 175–183. [CrossRef] [PubMed]
46. Jerse, A.E.; Sharma, N.D.; Simms, A.N.; Crow, E.T.; Snyder, L.A.; Shafer, W.M. A gonococcal efflux pump system enhances bacterial survival in a female mouse model of genital tract infection. *Infect. Immun.* **2003**, *71*, 5576–5582. [CrossRef] [PubMed]
47. Rouquette, C.; Harmon, J.B.; Shafer, W.M. Induction of the mtrCDE-encoded efflux pump system of Neisseria gonorrhoeae requires MtrA, an AraC-like protein. *Mol. Microbiol.* **1999**, *33*, 651–658. [CrossRef] [PubMed]
48. Xiao, L.; Crabb, D.M.; Dai, Y.; Chen, Y.; Waites, K.B.; Atkinson, T.P. Suppression of antimicrobial peptide expression by ureaplasma species. *Infect. Immun.* **2014**, *82*, 1657–1665. [CrossRef]
49. Zughaier, S.M. Neisseria meningitidis capsular polysaccharides induce inflammatory responses via TLR2 and TLR4-MD-2. *J. Leukoc. Biol.* **2011**, *89*, 469–480. [CrossRef]

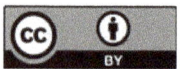

© 2020 by the authors. Licensee MDPI, Basel, Switzerland. This article is an open access article distributed under the terms and conditions of the Creative Commons Attribution (CC BY) license (http://creativecommons.org/licenses/by/4.0/).

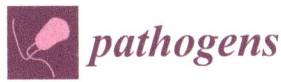

Article

Can Ciprofloxacin be Used for Precision Treatment of Gonorrhea in Public STD Clinics? Assessment of Ciprofloxacin Susceptibility and an Opportunity for Point-of-Care Testing

Johan H. Melendez [1,*], Yu-Hsiang Hsieh [2], Mathilda Barnes [1], Justin Hardick [1], Elizabeth A. Gilliams [3] and Charlotte A. Gaydos [1]

[1] Division of Infectious Diseases, Johns Hopkins School of Medicine, Baltimore, MD 21205, USA; mbarnes2@jhmi.edu (M.B.); jhardic1@jhmi.edu (J.H.); cgaydos@jhmi.edu (C.A.G.)
[2] Department of Emergency Medicine, Johns Hopkins University, Baltimore, MD 21205, USA; yhsieh1@jhmi.edu
[3] Johns Hopkins School of Medicine, Baltimore, MD 21205, USA; Elizabeth.Gilliams@baltimorecity.gov
* Correspondence: jmelend3@jhmi.edu

Received: 18 September 2019; Accepted: 4 October 2019; Published: 14 October 2019

Abstract: Background: Given the lack of new antimicrobials to treat *Neisseria gonorrhoeae* (NG) infections, reusing previously recommended antimicrobials has been proposed as a strategy to control the spread of multi-drug-resistant NG. We assessed ciprofloxacin susceptibility in a large sample set of NG isolates and identified correlates associated with ciprofloxacin-resistant NG infections. **Methods**: NG isolates collected in Baltimore, Maryland between 2014 and 2016 were evaluated by Gyrase A (*gyrA*) PCR and E-test for susceptibility to ciprofloxacin. Clinical characteristics and demographics were evaluated by multivariate regression analysis to identify correlates of ciprofloxacin-resistant NG infections. **Results**: 510 NG isolates from predominately African American (96.5%), heterosexual (85.7%), and HIV-negative (92.5%) male subjects were included in the study. The overall percentage of isolates with mutant *gyrA* sequences, indicative of ciprofloxacin resistance, was 32.4%, and significantly increased from 24.7% in 2014 to 45.2% in 2016 ($p < 0.001$). Participants older than 35 years of age were 2.35 times more likely to have a *gyrA* mutant NG infection than younger participants ($p < 0.001$). Race, sexual orientation, symptomology, or co-infection the HIV or syphilis were not associated with a particular NG *gyrA* genotype. **Conclusions**: Resistance to ciprofloxacin in Baltimore is lower than other regions and indicates that in this environment, use of ciprofloxacin may be appropriate for targeted treatment provided utilization of enhanced surveillance tools. The targeted use of ciprofloxacin may be more beneficial for individuals under 35 years of age. Point-of-care tests for NG diagnosis and susceptibility testing are urgently needed to identify individuals who can be treated with this targeted approach.

Keywords: *Neisseria gonorrhoeae*; gonorrhea; antimicrobial resistance; ciprofloxacin resistance; precision treatment

1. Introduction

Gonorrhea is the second most prevalent bacterial sexually transmitted infection (STI) worldwide, with an estimated 87 million infections in 2016 [1]. In the United States, 555,608 cases of gonorrhea were reported to the Centers for Disease Control and Prevention (CDC) in 2017, a 67% increase from 2013 [2]. *Neisseria gonorrhoeae* (NG) has progressively developed resistance to all commonly-prescribed antimicrobials [3] and is considered as one of the top three urgent threats among antibiotic-resistant bacteria [4].

In response to the threat of multidrug-resistant NG, the World Health Organization (WHO) has proposed a global action plan, comprising several strategies, to mitigate the emergence and spread of antimicrobial resistant (AMR) NG [5]. One of the strategies proposed by the WHO to combat AMR NG is the development of molecular methodologies for monitoring and detecting antimicrobial resistance in NG. Traditionally, the determination of AMR NG has been performed by minimum inhibitory concentration (MIC) testing, which requires viable organisms for proper execution. A well developed and validated molecular method for AMR determination could obviate the requirement for a viable clinical isolate. It has been hypothesized that antimicrobial susceptibility testing (AST) at the point-of-care (POC) could lead to precision treatment, i.e., utilizing specific antibiotics based on the AMR profile of NG as opposed to syndromic management of NG infections, including reusing previously recommended antimicrobials. This approach could reduce ceftriaxone selection pressure as ceftriaxone is one of the few remaining antibiotics effective against NG, and help delay the emergence of extended spectrum cephalosporin (ESC) resistance or untreatable gonorrhea [6,7].

Ciprofloxacin, a previously recommended antimicrobial, is an excellent candidate for precision treatment as 69.9% of NG isolates collected by the gonococcal isolate surveillance project (GISP) in 2017 were susceptible to ciprofloxacin [8]. Furthermore, ciprofloxacin susceptibility can be reliably predicted through the detection of genetic markers, thus allowing for the characterization of ciprofloxacin susceptibility directly from a variety of clinical specimens, including those used for the nucleic acid amplification test (NAAT)-based detection of gonorrhea [9]. At the molecular level, resistance to ciprofloxacin is strongly associated with a single mutation at codon 91 of the *gyrase A* (*gyrA*) gene [10], and detection of this mutation has been shown to be an excellent predictor of ciprofloxacin resistance [9,10]. Although other codons in *gyrA*, as well as in topoisomerase IV (*parC*), and in rare instances, penicillin binding protein 2 (PBP2/*PenA*) have been associated with resistance to ciprofloxacin, the vast majority of ciprofloxacin-resistant NG harbor the single mutation at codon 91 of *GyrA*, making this gene the target of choice for molecular screening [3,9]. As such, in 2016, a health care-based system study showed that implementation of a single molecular assay testing for *gyrA* mutations could be utilized in clinical care, and reduced the use of ceftriaxone while increasing the use of ciprofloxacin [11]. Furthermore, patients with wildtype *gyrA* NG who were treated with ciprofloxacin successfully cleared the infection at all anatomical sites of infections [12]. Despite the successful use of ciprofloxacin in clinical settings, this approach has not been evaluated in STI clinic settings, where this approach could potentially be highly effective.

Baltimore, Maryland, a large city with a high prevalence of gonorrhea (691.7/100,000 in 2017) [13], could be an excellent setting for the re-use of ciprofloxacin as a treatment option. According to our previous study, over 55% of the NG isolates collected in 2016 were susceptible to ciprofloxacin [14]. However, additional studies are necessary to better define the epidemiology of ciprofloxacin-resistant NG in Baltimore and determine whether ciprofloxacin could be effectively re-used in this particular population. In this study, we report the epidemiology of ciprofloxacin resistance in Baltimore through the molecular analysis of 510 NG isolates collected between 2014 and 2016. Additionally, clinical characteristics and demographics were evaluated to identify correlates of ciprofloxacin-resistant NG infections.

2. Results

A total of 510 urethral NG isolates collected from 2014 to 2016 were included in the study. The isolates were recovered from 510 male subjects (15–69 years old), predominately African American (96.5%), heterosexual (85.7%), and HIV-uninfected (92.5%) (Table 1). The majority of participants (96.7%) reported symptoms of urethritis at the time of sample of collection, and 4.3% were co-infected with syphilis.

Table 1. Characteristics of 510 men with *Neisseria gonorrhoeae* infection in Baltimore, 2014–2016.

Characteristics	Categories	Number (%)
		N = 510
Age (Years)	15–19	60 (11.8)
	20–24	117 (22.9)
	25–29	109 (21.4)
	30–34	57 (11.2)
	35–44	85 (16.7)
	≥45	82 (16.1)
Race/Ethnicity	African American	492 (96.5)
	Non-Hispanic White	11 (2.2)
	Hispanic	3 (0.6)
	Other	4 (0.8)
Sexual Orientation	Heterosexual	437 (85.7)
	Bisexual	17 (3.3)
	Gay	50 (9.8)
	Unknown/Unspecified	6 (1.2)
Calendar Year	2014	170 (33.3)
	2015	185 (36.3)
	2016	155 (30.4)
Symptoms	Discharge	459 (90.0)
	Dysuria	253 (49.6)
	Itch in urogenital area	19 (3.7)
	Lesion in urogenital area	16 (3.1)
	Irritation or tingling feeling	13 (2.5)
	Burning sensation	7 (1.4)
	Rash	6 (1.2)
	Pain in urogenital area	5 (1.0)
	Other	2 (0.4)
	None	17 (3.3)
HIV Infection	Yes	34 (6.7)
	No	472 (92.5)
	Unknown	4 (0.8)
Concurrent Syphilis Infection	Yes	22 (4.3)
	No	488 (95.7)
Syphilis Diagnosis in the Past	Yes	25 (4.9)
	No	485 (95.1)
GyrA Genotype	Wild type	345 (67.7)
	Mutant	165 (32.4)

The number of isolates collected by year was uniformly distributed: 170 (33.3%), 185 (36.3%), and 155 (30.4%), collected in 2014, 2015, and 2016, respectively. Genotypic typing by PCR revealed that 32.4% (165/510) of the isolates had mutation(s) in the *gyrA* gene. The percentage of isolates with *gyrA* mutant sequences was 24.7% (42/170), 28.7% (53/185), and 45.2% (70/155) in 2014, 2015, and 2016, respectively. The increase in the percentage of *gyrA* mutant NG from 2014 to 2016 was statistically significant ($p < 0.001$) in a bivariate and multivariate regression analysis (Tables 2 and 3). Multivariate analysis was specifically used to determine the predictor of our outcomes adjusted for co-variates period of the 165 NG isolates with mutant *gyrA* sequences; 63.6% (105/165) were viable for susceptibility testing, and 98.1% (103/105) were confirmed as ciprofloxacin resistant by the E-test method. The remaining two isolates displayed intermediate resistance to ciprofloxacin. Susceptibility testing of 92 randomly selected isolates with *gyrA* wildtype sequences showed that all isolates were susceptible to ciprofloxacin.

Table 2. Bivariate analysis of association between demographic and clinical characteristics and *gyrA* genotype among 510 men with *Neisseria gonorrhoeae* infection in Baltimore, 2014–2016.

Characteristics	Categories	*gyrA* Genotype Wild Type N = 345	*gyrA* Genotype Mutant N = 165	p-Value
Age (Years)*	15–24	135 (39.1)	42 (25.5)	0.002
	25–34	113 (32.8)	53 (32.1)	
	≥35	97 (28.1)	70 (42.4)	
Race/Ethnicity	African American	334 (96.8)	158 (95.8)	0.546
Sexual Orientation	Bisexual or Gay	51 (14.8)	16 (9.7)	0.112
Calendar Year†	2014	128 (37.1)	42 (25.5)	<0.001
	2015	132 (38.3)	53 (32.1)	
	2016	85 (24.6)	70 (42.4)	
Symptom—Discharge	Discharge	312 (90.4)	147 (89.1)	0.636
Symptom—Dysuria	Dysuria	176 (51.0)	77 (46.7)	0.358
No Symptom	Yes	9 (2.6)	8 (4.9)	0.187
HIV Infection	Yes	26 (7.5)	8 (4.9)	0.255
Concurrent Syphilis Infection	Yes	15 (4.4)	7 (4.2)	0.956
Syphilis Diagnosis in the Past	Yes	16 (4.6)	9 (5.5)	0.689

* $p < 0.001$ for Cochran–Armitage Trend Test; † $p < 0.001$ for Cochran–Armitage Trend Test.

Table 3. Multivariate regression analysis of factors associated with presence of *gyrA* genotype among 510 men with *Neisseria gonorrhoeae* infection in Baltimore, 2014–2016.

Variables	Categories	Odds Ratio (95% CI)	p-Value
Age Group (years)	15–24	1.00	
	25–34	1.46 (0.90, 2.37)	0.123
	≥35	2.35 (1.47, 3.76)	<0.001
Calendar Year	Increasing each year	1.61 (1.27, 2.05)	<0.001

Stratification of the isolates by *gyrA* genotype revealed that older age was associated with a mutant *gyrA* genotype ($p = 0.002$), suggestive of an association between ciprofloxacin resistance and age (Table 2), and participants ≥35 years of age were 2.35 times (95% CI, 1.47–3.76) more likely to have a *gyrA* mutant NG infection than younger participants ($p < 0.001$) (Table 3). Race, sexual orientation, symptomology, or co-infection with another STI (HIV or syphilis) were not associated with a particular NG *gyrA* genotype (Table 2).

3. Discussion

As the first step in the development of a POC test for gonorrhea diagnosis and antimicrobial susceptibility testing, we sought to determine whether ciprofloxacin could be a suitable antimicrobial for precision treatment in Baltimore. Using a molecular approach, we have shown low to moderate levels of ciprofloxacin resistance in Baltimore during a three-year period, suggesting that this antimicrobial might be a suitable option for precision treatment. Furthermore, our study identified an association between age and ciprofloxacin-resistant NG infections.

The overall percentage (32.4%) of mutant *gyrA* NG infections, and thus resistance to ciprofloxacin, in our study is similar to the nationwide percentage (30.1%) reported by GISP in 2017 [8]. The high percentage of wildtype *gyrA* (ciprofloxacin-susceptible) NG isolates in this study provides further evidence for the use of ciprofloxacin for targeted precision treatment, which may help to delay the emergence and spread of resistance to current first-line regimens [6,7]. Additionally, use of ciprofloxacin could make partner therapy easier. However, the increase in the percentage of isolates with mutated *gyrA* sequences from 2014 to 2016 (24.7 to 45.2%), which is consistent with national trends [15], suggests that ciprofloxacin resistance has persisted despite ciprofloxacin not being used as a recommended treatment option for gonorrhea. Therefore, the reintroduction of ciprofloxacin as a gonorrhea treatment option will require enhanced surveillance practices to determine if and when the targeted treatment is no longer a viable option.

Our study also identified age as an important demographic correlate associated with ciprofloxacin-resistant NG infections. Men older than 35 years of age were 2.35 times more likely to have a mutant *gyrA* NG infection than younger men. On the contrary, men under 24 years of age were more likely to have a wildtype *gyrA* (ciprofloxacin-susceptible) infection. These findings suggest that younger individuals (<24 years of age) may be the ideal population for targeted precision treatment with ciprofloxacin. A targeted treatment approach may prove efficacious in older individuals, but caution is warranted considering the higher percentage of ciprofloxacin resistance observed in this study and the results of previous studies which have reported an association between older age and antimicrobial-resistant NG infections [16]. Contrary to previous studies [16], our study did not find an association between ciprofloxacin-resistant NG and sexual orientation; however, the number of NG isolates from men who have sex with men (MSM) was limited, and a larger study focusing on MSM may provide more details.

The re-introduction of ciprofloxacin as a treatment option could help to mitigate the emergence and spread of AMR NG. According to a modeling study, the introduction of a POC ciprofloxacin susceptibility test could help to decrease the use of ceftriaxone by as much as 66%, thus potentially helping to extend the usefulness of this antimicrobial [17]. However, caution is warranted since the introduction of a POC test targeting a single antimicrobial, such as ciprofloxacin, may accelerate the emergence of triply-resistant (ciprofloxacin, ceftriaxone, and azithromycin) NG isolates [7]. These modelling studies highlight the need for the development of POC tests for resistance to multiple antimicrobials, but the complex resistance mechanisms of other antimicrobials, such as ceftriaxone [3], have hindered the development of such molecular tests. Phenotypic tests, on the other hand, may determine resistance to multiple antimicrobials, but are not currently available at the POC. Therefore, until POC tests targeting multiple antimicrobials can be developed, a single antimicrobial POC test, capable of providing an alternative treatment option, such as ciprofloxacin, might be the most suitable option. The development of a POC test for gonorrhea and identification of ciprofloxacin susceptibility is attractive because ciprofloxacin can be administered before the patient leaves the clinic.

Our study had several limitations. First, all of the isolates were collected in Baltimore, Maryland at one clinic, thus limiting the generalizability and scope of these results. However, the data reported by GISP in 2017 suggest low levels of ciprofloxacin resistance in the US [8]. Second, we had limited access to epidemiological, complete demographic, and behavioral data, which limited the scope of our analysis. It should also be noted that these samples were collected between 2014 and 2016; it is likely that the levels of ciprofloxacin susceptibility and resistance have varied since then, and these results should be viewed with that caveat. Finally, samples from women and samples from extragenital sites (pharyngeal and rectal) were not available for this analysis. Additionally, a more complete approach to the study would have been to expand molecular testing to include *ParC* targets associated with ciprofloxacin resistance, as well as the rare *PenA* target associated with ciprofloxacin resistance. However, as stated previously, the vast majority of ciprofloxacin-resistant NG harbor the single mutation at codon 91 of *GyrA*, and focusing on this target, as similar studies have shown, proves to be just as effective at identifying ciprofloxacin susceptibility and resistance, as expanded tests show.

4. Conclusions

In conclusion, we have shown that a large proportion of the NG isolates tested in this study are susceptible to ciprofloxacin, providing further support for the use of this antimicrobial for targeted treatment if ciprofloxacin susceptibility can be determined at the POC. Current treatment guidelines for NG from multiple health organizations state that ceftriaxone (CRO) plus azithromycin (AZM), or cefixime (CFX), are the standards, but these guidelines are based on a syndromic approach to disease management [3,5]. Given the overall increase in resistance to multiple classes of antibiotics, syndromic management of NG may no longer be the most appropriate strategy. Even in this study, the increase in resistance during the study period highlights the need for continued and improved surveillance practices. Given the lower proportion of ciprofloxacin resistance in younger individuals, a targeted surveillance approach may be more beneficial for patients under 35 years of age as it increases the likelihood of identifying ciprofloxacin susceptible NG. Additional studies aimed at identifying facilitators and potential barriers towards the implementation of POC susceptibility testing and precision treatment in the STI clinic setting are warranted.

5. Materials and Methods

5.1. Clinical Data

This study was approved by the Johns Hopkins University School of Medicine Institutional Review Board. For purposes of statistical analysis to determine potential risk factors and clinical correlates associated with acquisition of ciprofloxacin-resistant NG, clinical data (age, race, sexual orientation, HIV status, current and past diagnosis of a Syphilis infection) were collected by record review.

5.2. NG Isolates

NG isolates were recovered from the urethra of symptomatic men seeking STI testing at the Baltimore City Health Department (BCHD) Druid Health Clinic from January 2014 to October 2016. Following culture, gram-negative diplococci, oxidase-positive bacterial isolates were presumptively classified as NG, stored in trypticase soy broth (TSB) with 20% glycerol, and frozen at −80 °C.

For this study, isolates were recovered by growth on chocolate agar plates incubated overnight in 5% CO_2 and the colonies re-suspended in phosphate buffered saline (PBS). Two-hundred microliters of each bacterial suspension was extracted for DNA using the automated MagNA Pure LC instrument (Roche Diagnostics, Indianapolis, IN, USA). Following DNA extraction, the isolates were confirmed as NG using a previously described PCR assay targeting the *opa* gene [18,19]. For non-viable isolates, 200 μL of the isolate-containing TSB media was extracted for total DNA as described above.

5.3. Molecular Characterization of Ciprofloxacin Susceptibility

In order to determine ciprofloxacin susceptibility at the molecular level, all isolates (viable and non-viable) were analyzed by real-time PCR for the presence/absence of mutation(s) in the *gyrA* gene using a previously described assay [19,20]. The PCR assay targets wildtype *gyrA* sequences, which are highly predictive of ciprofloxacin susceptibility [9]. NG isolates with negative *gyrA* PCR results were classified as *gyrA* mutant, which is indicative of ciprofloxacin resistance.

5.4. Antimicrobial Susceptibility Testing

All viable NG isolates with mutated *gyrA* sequences were further analyzed by the E-test method, (bioMérieux, Durham, NC, USA), to determine the minimum inhibitory concentration (MIC) of ciprofloxacin, as we previously described [14]. Additionally, all viable NG isolates with wildtype *gyrA* sequences, collected in 2016, and a subset of isolates collected in 2014 were also tested using the E-test method. Phenotypic susceptibility testing on isolates collected in 2015 was not performed, because none of those isolates were viable for analysis. Briefly, bacterial suspensions, matching a 0.5

MacFarland standard, were plated on GC agar medium (Becton Dickinson, Sparks, MD, USA) media supplemented with 1% IsoVitaleX (Becton Dickinson, Franklin Lakes, NJ, USA) and allowed to air dry for 5 minutes. E-test strips containing ciprofloxacin were individually placed on the inoculated agar surface according to manufacturer's recommendations, incubated at 37 °C in a moist 5% CO_2-enriched environment, and MIC results recorded after 18–24 h. The MIC was determined by reading the intercept of the inhibition zone and the E-test strip. Breakpoints for ciprofloxacin resistance were selected in accordance with guidelines set forth by the Clinical and Laboratory Standards Institute (CLSI) [21].

5.5. Statistical Analysis

Bivariate analysis was performed using the chi-square test. The Cochran–Armitage Trend test was performed to evaluate yearly trends. The multivariate model was used to determine the predictor of our outcomes adjusted for co-variates. In this case, age group was the key predictor, and we strongly believed that calendar years and others could be either covariates for the outcomes. Therefore, we built this full model first, then used multivariate analysis to identify the final model. The final model was built in a stepwise manner. All analyses were conducted using SAS version 9.4

Author Contributions: J.H.M., J.H., and C.A.G. contributed to the conception and design of the study. J.H.M. and J.H. contributed to analysis and interpretation of data. Y.-H.H. performed statistical analyses. E.A.G. contributed to collecting the *Neisseria gonorrhoeae* isolates. J.H.M. and M.B. contributed to collecting the data. J.H.M., J.H., and C.A.G drafted the manuscript. All authors reviewed and approved the final manuscript.

Funding: This research was funded by the National Institutes of Health (NIBIB 1U54 EB007958) and (NIAID U-01068613).

Conflicts of Interest: The authors declare no conflict of interest.

References

1. Rowley, J.; Vander Hoorn, S.; Korenromp, E.; Low, N.; Unemo, M.; Abu-Raddad, L.J.; Chico, R.M.; Smolak, A.; Newman, L.; Gottlieb, S.; et al. Chlamydia, gonorrhoea, trichomoniasis and syphilis: Global prevalence and incidence estimates, 2016. *Bull. World Health Organ.* **2019**, *97*, 548–562. [CrossRef] [PubMed]
2. Centers for Disease Control and Prevention. *Sexually Transmitted Disease Surveillance 2017*; U.S. Department of Health and Human Services: Atlanta, GA, USA, 2017. Available online: https://www.cdc.gov/std/stats17/default.htm (accessed on 20 May 2019).
3. Unemo, M.; Del Rio, C.; Shafer, W.M. Antimicrobial Resistance Expressed by *Neisseria gonorrhoeae*: A Major Global Public Health Problem in the 21st Century. *Microbiol. Spectr.* **2016**, *4*, 1–10. [CrossRef] [PubMed]
4. Centers for Disease Control and Prevention. 2013. Antibiotic Resistance Threats in the United States. CDC, US Department of Health and Human Services. Available online: https://www.cdc.gov/drugresistance/pdf/ar-threats-2013-508.pdf (accessed on 10 May 2019).
5. WHO 2012. Global Action Plan to Control the Spread and Impact of Antimicrobial Resistance in Neisseria gonorrhoeae. Available online: http://www.who.int/reproductivehealth/publications/rtis/9789241503501/en/ (accessed on 25 October 2018).
6. Sadiq, S.T.; Mazzaferri, F.; Unemo, M. Rapid accurate point-of-care tests combining diagnostics and antimicrobial resistance prediction for *Neisseria gonorrhoeae* and *Mycoplasma genitalium*. *Sex. Transm. Infect.* **2017**, *93*, S63–S68. [CrossRef] [PubMed]
7. Tuite, A.R.; Gift, T.L.; Chesson, H.W.; Hsu, K.; Salomon, J.A.; Grad, Y.H. Impact of rapid susceptibility testing and antibiotic selection strategy on the emergence and spread of antibiotic resistance in gonorrhea. *J. Infect. Dis.* **2017**, *216*, 1141–1149. [CrossRef] [PubMed]
8. Centers for Disease Control and Prevention. Gonococcal Isolate Surveillance Project (GISP) Profiles. 2017. Available online: https://www.cdc.gov/std/stats17/GISP2017/default.htm (accessed on 20 May 2019).
9. Allan-Blitz, L.T.; Wang, X.; Klausner, J.D. Wild-Type Gyrase A Genotype of *Neisseria gonorrhoeae* Predicts In Vitro Susceptibility to Ciprofloxacin: A Systematic Review of the Literature and Meta-Analysis. *Sex. Transm. Dis.* **2017**, *44*, 261–265. [CrossRef] [PubMed]

10. Belland, R.J.; Morrison, S.G.; Ison, C.; Huang, W.M. *Neisseria gonorrhoeae* acquires mutations in analogous regions of *gyrA* and *parC* in fluoroquinolone resistant isolates. *Mol. Microbiol.* **1994**, *14*, 371–380. [CrossRef] [PubMed]
11. Allan-Blitz, L.T.; Humphries, R.M.; Hemarajata, P.; Bhatti, A.; Pandori, M.W.; Siedner, M.J.; Klausner, J.D. Implementation of a Rapid Genotypic Assay to Promote Targeted Ciprofloxacin Therapy of *Neisseria gonorrhoeae* in a Large Health System. *Clin. Infect. Dis.* **2017**, *64*, 1268–1270. [CrossRef] [PubMed]
12. Allan-Blitz, L.T.; Hemarajata, P.; Humphries, R.M.; Kimble, M.; Elias, S.; Klausner, J.D. Ciprofloxacin May be Efficacious in Treating Wild-Type *Gyrase A* Genotype *Neisseria gonorrhoeae* Infections. *Sex. Transm. Dis.* **2018**, *45*, e18. [CrossRef] [PubMed]
13. Center for Sexually Transmitted Infection Prevention. Division of Hygiene and Mental health. Baltimore City Health Department; Maryland Office of Planning. 2017. Available online: https://phpa.health.maryland.gov/OIDPCS/CSTIP/Pages/STI-Data-Statistics.aspx (accessed on 25 June 2018).
14. Melendez, J.H.; Hardick, J.; Barnes, M.; Page, K.R.; Gaydos, C.A. Antimicrobial Susceptibility of *Neisseria gonorrhoeae* Isolates in Baltimore, Maryland, 2016: The Importance of Sentinel Surveillance in the Era of Multi-Drug-Resistant Gonorrhea. *Antibiotics* **2018**, *7*, 77. [CrossRef] [PubMed]
15. St. Cyr, S.; Torrone, E.; Workowski, K. As a response to STD treatment guideline updates, have *Neisseria gonorrhoeae* strains regained susceptibility to ciprofloxacin? *Sex. Transm. Dis.* **2018**, *45*, S39.
16. Abraha, M.; Egli-Gany, D.; Low, N. Epidemiological, behavioural, and clinical factors associated with antimicrobial-resistant gonorrhoea: A review. *F1000Research* **2018**, *7*, 400. [CrossRef] [PubMed]
17. Turner, K.M.; Christensen, H.; Adams, E.J.; McAdams, D.; Fifer, H.; McDonnell, A.; Woodford, N. Analysis of the potential for point-of-care test to enable individualised treatment of infections caused by antimicrobial-resistant and susceptible strains of *Neisseria gonorrhoeae*: A modelling study. *BMJ Open* **2017**, *7*, e015447. [CrossRef] [PubMed]
18. Tabrizi, S.N.; Chen, S.; Tapsall, J.; Garlan, S.M. Evaluation of opa-based real-time PCR for detection of *Neisseria gonorrhoeae*. *Sex. Transm. Dis.* **2005**, *32*, 199–202. [CrossRef] [PubMed]
19. Melendez, J.H.; Hardick, J.; Barnes, M.; Barnes, P.; Geddes, C.D. Gaydos, C.A. Molecular Characterization of Markers Associated with Antimicrobial Resistance in *Neisseria gonorrhoeae* Identified from Residual Clinical Samples. *Sex. Transm. Dis.* **2018**, *45*, 312–315. [CrossRef] [PubMed]
20. Giles, J.; Hardick, J.; Yuenger, J.; Dan, M.; Reich, K.; Zenilman, J. Use of applied biosystems 7900HT sequence detection system and TaqMan assay for detection of quinolone-resistant *Neisseria gonorrhoeae*. *J. Clin. Microbiol.* **2004**, *42*, 3281–3283. [CrossRef] [PubMed]
21. Clinical and Laboratory Standard Institute. *Performance Standards for Antimicrobial Susceptibility Testing*, 28th ed.; CLSI supplement M100; CLSI: Wayne, PA, USA, 2018.

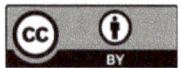

© 2019 by the authors. Licensee MDPI, Basel, Switzerland. This article is an open access article distributed under the terms and conditions of the Creative Commons Attribution (CC BY) license (http://creativecommons.org/licenses/by/4.0/).

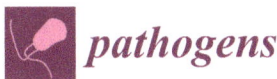

Review

To What Extent Should We Rely on Antibiotics to Reduce High Gonococcal Prevalence? Historical Insights from Mass-Meningococcal Campaigns

Chris Kenyon [1,2]

[1] HIV/STI Unit, Institute of Tropical Medicine, 2000 Antwerp, Belgium; kenyon@itg.be; Tel.: +32-3-2480796; Fax: +32-3-2480831

[2] Division of Infectious Diseases and HIV Medicine, University of Cape Town, Anzio Road, Observatory 7700, South Africa

Received: 15 January 2020; Accepted: 17 February 2020; Published: 18 February 2020

Abstract: In the absence of a vaccine, current antibiotic-dependent efforts to reduce the prevalence of *Neisseria gonorrhoeae* in high prevalence populations have been shown to result in extremely high levels of antibiotic consumption. No randomized controlled trials have been conducted to validate this strategy and an important concern of this approach is that it may induce antimicrobial resistance. To contribute to this debate, we assessed if mass treatment in the related species, *Neisseria meningitidis*, was associated with the emergence of antimicrobial resistance. To this end, we conducted a historical review of the effect of mass meningococcal treatment programmes on the prevalence of *N. meningitidis* and the emergence of antimicrobial resistance. We found evidence that mass treatment programmes were associated with the emergence of antimicrobial resistance.

Keywords: *Neisseria gonorrhoeae*; AMR; *Neisseria meningitides*; commensal Neisseria

1. Introduction

The World Health Organization's plan to reduce the incidence of *Neisseria (N.) gonorrhoeae* by 90% by 2030 faces two growing challenges—antimicrobial resistance and rising rather than falling incidence of *N. gonorrhoeae* in many key populations [1,2]. A number of the strategies advocated to reduce gonococcal incidence such as intensified screening, partner tracing/expedited partner therapy and doxycycline pre-exposure prophylaxis, depend on increasing antibiotic consumption [2,3]. These increases can be large. Screening for gonorrhoea/chlamydia at three sites every three months in HIV pre-exposure prophylaxis (PrEP) cohorts, for example, has been shown to result in very large macrolide and cephalosporin exposures. Macrolide exposure, for example, can reach 4400 defined daily doses/1000 population per year, which is approximately 20 times the population consumption of a country such as Sweden [4]. A concern of such high levels of antibiotic consumption is the induction of antimicrobial resistance (AMR) in *N. gonorrhoeae* and other organisms [4].

To assist in the evaluation of this concern, we undertook a historical review of the effect of mass antimicrobial treatments on antimicrobial susceptibility of the related *Neisseria*, *N. meningitidis.* There have been few mass treatment trials of *N. gonorrhoeae*. These studies have typically found that mass treatment has no effect [5–7], or only a temporary effect on gonorrhoea incidence/prevalence [8,9]. Only one of these studies evaluated the effect on AMR. Although this study found a temporal association between mass treatment and the emergence of gonococcal AMR, its contemporary relevance is reduced by the fact that it was conducted using penicillin in the 1960s [8,9].

Considerably more mass treatment studies have been conducted for *N. meningitidis*. These mass treatment studies involved the widespread administration of antibiotic therapy (chemoprophylaxis) to a community with either excess cases of meningococcal disease or a raised prevalence of asymptomatic *N. meningitidis* [10–13].

Although there are important differences in the mode of transmission, preferred site of colonization, clinical presentation and host immune response between *N. meningitidis* and *N. gonorrhoeae*, there are also considerable similarities [14,15]. Despite being the only two species in the *Neisseria* genus that are classified as strict human pathogens, the majority of both infections are asymptomatic and resolve spontaneously. Both infections cluster in particular population groups. In the case of meningococcus, and in keeping with its respiratory transmission, epidemics and high carriage rates are predominantly associated with young adults living in crowded conditions [11–13]. *N. gonorrhoeae* is sexually transmitted and thus a high prevalence has been linked to factors such as high rates of sexual partner turnover which generate dense sexual networks and high equilibrium prevalences of *N. gonorrhoeae* [2,16–19]. In the case of PrEP cohorts, for example, modelling studies suggest that the five to ten sexual partners per three months reported by PrEP recipients generate the high prevalence of *N. gonorrhoeae* in these populations—typically around 10% [16,20]. Crucially, the two infections are genotypically closely related and able to exchange DNA between one another and commensal *Neisseria* via well-developed systems of transformation [21–23]. The uptake of DNA from other *Neisseria* species has been established as a key way that both the gono- and meningococcus have acquired antimicrobial resistance [21–23]. *N. gonorrhoeae* has been noted to be more susceptible to the emergence of AMR than *N. meningitidis* [24]. These considerations suggest that if mass treatment of *N. meningitidis* is associated with the emergence of AMR, this would provide a cautionary warning for using antibiotic based strategies to reduce the prevalence of *N. gonorrhoeae* in high prevalence settings such as PrEP cohorts.

2. Effect of Mass Treatment on Prevalence of *N. meningitidis*, Meningitis Cases and AMR

A recent review paper by MacNamara et al. evaluated the effect of mass treatment of *N. meningitidis* on the prevalence of the bacteria and the emergence of AMR in over 33 studies [10]. The authors concluded that the intervention was highly effective in reducing cases of meningitis and, when an effective antibiotic was used at over 75% population coverage, this resulted in a 50% to 80% reduction in carriage in the short term (median follow up six weeks). In the one study with less than 75% coverage, there was no reduction in carriage [25]. This review paper did not evaluate the long-term effects. One of the few studies to assess this was a study from a Kibbutz, in Israel, that found that mass treatment resulted in a decline in carriage but this effect only lasted six months [26].

Although the effect on AMR was not assessed in all studies, when it was assessed, AMR emerged fairly frequently. Resistance to rifampicin was particularly evident and found in all three community studies where this was assessed [10,25,27,28]. Rifampicin resistance was also noted in cases following two mass therapy interventions in the United States of America (US) military [10]. Sulfadiazine was used extensively in the US military to prevent meningococcal disease from the 1940s to the 1960s [29]. This widespread use was thought to play a role in the rapid and extensive emergence of AMR in the 1950s and 1960s [29]. Only one study tested for ciprofloxacin resistance following use of this agent. This study found no ciprofloxacin resistance but only evaluated for resistance six months after the intervention [30]. No studies evaluated the emergence of resistance to other antimicrobials such as ceftriaxone and azithromycin.

2.1. Individual Level Assessment

A systematic review of the efficacy of various antibiotics for the eradication of *N. meningitidis* carriage found that penicillin, rifampicin, minocycline, ciprofloxacin and ceftriaxone were effective at eradicating carriage for up to four weeks [31]. Eleven trials reported the susceptibility of persistent isolates to the antibiotic used for elimination. Six of these studies evaluated the induction of AMR by rifampicin. Resistance was found in persistent isolates in three of these six studies—the prevalence of resistance was between 10% and 27% [31]. The use of other antibiotics was not associated with the selection of resistance.

2.2. Association between Overcrowding and N. meningitidis Prevalence/outbreaks

We could not find any systematic reviews on this topic, but there was broad consensus in the literature we reviewed that overcrowding (particularly for young adults) played a crucial role in outbreaks of meningococcal disease and increases in prevalence [11,13,26,32]. Glover was the first to describe this association in 1917 in an outbreak of meningococcal disease in soldiers in military recruitment camps. Using nasopharyngeal cultures to evaluate meningococcal colonization prevalence, he noted a steep increase in prevalence following the overcrowding of recruits (Figure 1) [13]. The camp was designed to accommodate 800 men but was accommodating close to 6000 men by the start of the epidemic. Of note, meningococcal prevalence decreased following measures that included reducing overcrowding (Figure 1). A range of subsequent studies and reviews of the topic have produced similar findings [11,26,32].

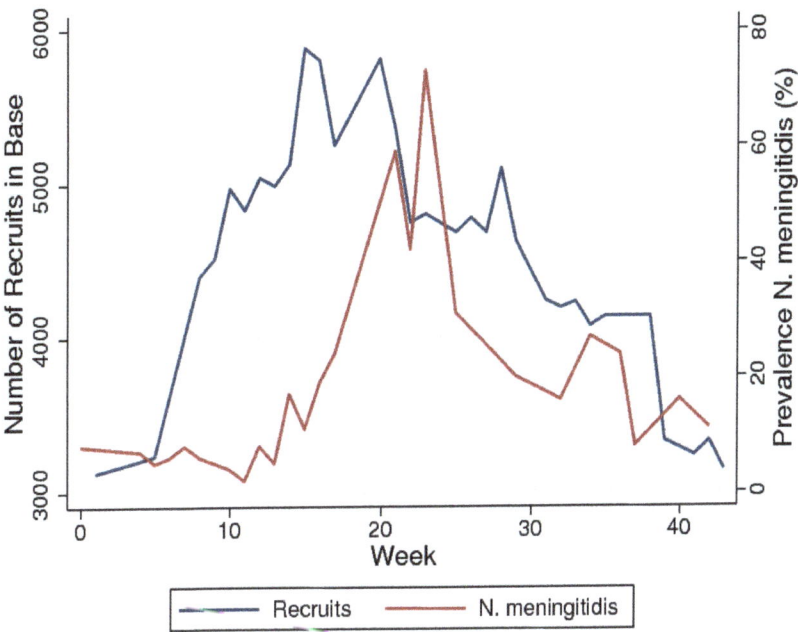

Figure 1. The temporal association between increased overcrowding (number of recruits) and prevalence of *N. meningitidis* in military recruits in a training camp in the south of England in 1917. Week 1 represents the first week of September 2017. (Based on data from [10] digitized with WebPlotDigitizer-4.2 and figure made in Stata 16.0).

3. Discussion

Mass treatment was fairly effective in the short term in reducing the prevalence of *N. meningitidis* but this effect did not appear to persist beyond six months. Mass treatments appeared to result in the emergence of AMR to rifampicin and sulphadiazine. There was little or no data for other classes of antibiotics.

The utility of these findings is limited by the fact that the effect of mass treatment with the antibiotics currently mostly used to treat *N. gonorrhoeae* (azithromycin/ceftriaxone) was not assessed. There are also important biological differences between *N. meningitidis* and *N. gonorrhoeae*, as well as differences between the mass administration of antibiotics during a meningococcal outbreak and the sustained high levels of antibiotic exposure in a PrEP cohort.

Despite these important reservations, the fact that AMR can emerge so rapidly in the related *N. meningitidis* does provide additional motivation to be alert for the emergence of gonococcal AMR in PrEP and other high antibiotic exposure populations. There is increasing evidence that horizontal gene transfer plays an important role in the genesis of AMR in *N. meningitidis* and even more so in *N. gonorrhoeae*. For example, it has been established that transformation from commensal pharyngeal *Neisseria* spp. played an important role in *N. gonorrhoeae's* acquisition of resistance to extended spectrum cephalosporins [33–35]. The acquisition of AMR via commensals can operate over much longer periods than direct selection during antibiotic therapy, as the commensals (and their resistance conferring genes) persist for longer periods than *N. gonorrhoeae*. These resistance genes can then be taken up months later by incoming gono- and meningococci [21–23]. We could not find any studies that evaluated the effect of mass treatments on the antibiotic susceptibility of commensal *Neisseria* species and, thus, we were unable to evaluate this effect. Unsurprisingly, however, studies have found a link between antibiotic susceptibility of commensal *Neisseria* and antibiotic consumption [36]. A study from Japan found high proportions of circulating *Neisseria subflava* to have high miminum inhibitory concentrations for penicillin, cefixime, ciprofloxacin and tetracycline [36]. This was thought to be related to the high levels of the corresponding antimicrobial consumed in Japan [36,37]. More direct evidence of this association comes from a study from Vietnam which found decreased cephalosporin susceptibility in commensal *Neisseria* to be related to recent cephalosporin consumption [38].

Two trials have been conducted to assess if doxycycline pre- and post-exposure could reduce the incidence of bacterial STIs including gonorrhoea [39,40]. Both studies found evidence of moderate reductions in chlamydia and syphilis incidence, but not gonorrhoea. The effect on AMR of pathogens and commensal organisms was not assessed in these studies.

Most people are persistently colonised during their lifetime with a variety of commensal *Neisseria* species, any of which can become a reservoir for AMR upon repeated exposure to antibiotic treatment of the host [41]. As a result, the selection pressure imposed by high antibiotic consumption is likely to be seen in these commensals before it becomes evident in gono- and menginococci [14]. As a result, commensal *Neisseria* could serve as an AMR early warning sign and it may be prudent to monitor the antibiotic susceptibilities of these commensal *Neisseria* species in high gonococcal prevalence and high antibiotic consumption populations, such as those on PrEP [42,43].

A further relevant parallel between gono- and meningococci is how the prevalence of both infections is strongly influenced by underlying dense contact networks—sexual networks and spatial networks, respectively [17–19]. It is these underlying networks which are thus primary determinants of high prevalence and should be the targets of radical prevention [19,43]. The high rates of partner change reported by PrEP recipients, for example, are responsible for the high prevalence of *N. gonorrhoeae* in this group [16,20]. This high network connectivity could be reduced by increased condom usage or reduced rates of partner turnover. Vaccination represents an enticing alternative strategy—as demonstrated by the efficacy of vaccination against *N. meningitidis* [44–49]. Although progress has been made in the development of a gonococcal vaccine, the best available vaccine (*N. meningitidis* group B outer membrane vaccine), appears to only have limited efficacy and for a short period [50–52]. In the absence of an effective vaccine, it is understandable that efforts to control increasing incidence of *N. gonorrhoeae* have focused on strategies relying on antibiotics. The evidence reviewed here suggests that extensive use of antibiotics to control *N. meningitidis* prevalence runs the risk of inducing AMR. These findings provide further justification to reconsider antibiotic based strategies to reduce gonococcal prevalence—such as three-monthly screening for gohorrhoea/chlamydia in PrEP cohorts. They also provide further motivation for enhanced surveillance of AMR in all *Neisseria* species in high prevalence, high antibiotic consumption populations.

Funding: No funding was received for this work.

Conflicts of Interest: The author declares no conflict of interest.

Abbreviations

AMR Antimicrobial resistance
PrEP Preexposure Prophylaxis
US   United States of America

References

1. World Health Organization. *Global Health Sector Strategy on Sexually Transmitted Infections 2016–2021*; Towards ending STIs; WHO: Geneva, Switzerland, 2016.
2. Unemo, M.; Bradshaw, C.S.; Hocking, J.S.; de Vries, H.J.C.; Francis, S.C.; Mabey, D.; Marrazzo, J.M.; Sonder, G.J.B.; Schwebke, J.R.; Hoornenborg, E.; et al. Sexually transmitted infections: Challenges ahead. *Lancet Infect. Dis.* **2017**, *17*, e235–e279. [CrossRef]
3. Kenyon, C.; Van Dijck, C.; Florence, E. Facing increased sexually transmitted infection incidence in HIV preexposure prophylaxis cohorts: What are the underlying determinants and what can be done? *Curr. Opin. Infect. Dis.* **2020**, *33*, 51–58. [CrossRef] [PubMed]
4. Kenyon, C. We need to consider collateral damage to resistomes when we decide how frequently to screen for chlamydia/gonorrhoea in PrEP cohorts. *AIDS* **2019**, *33*, 155–157. [CrossRef] [PubMed]
5. Wawer, M.J.; Sewankambo, N.K.; Serwadda, D.; Quinn, T.C.; Kiwanuka, N.; Li, C.; Lutalo, T.; Nalugoda, F.; Gaydos, C.A.; Moulton, L.H.; et al. Control of sexually transmitted diseases for AIDS prevention in Uganda: A randomised community trial. *Lancet* **1999**, *353*, 525–535. [CrossRef]
6. Wawer, M.J.; Gray, R.H.; Sewankambo, N.K.; Serwadda, D.; Paxton, L.; Berkley, S.; McNairn, D.; Wabwire-Mangen, F.; Li, C.; Nalugoda, F.; et al. A randomized, community trial of intensive sexually transmitted disease control for AIDS prevention, Rakai, Uganda. *AIDS* **1998**, *12*, 1211–1225. [CrossRef]
7. Ghys, P.D.; Diallo, M.O.; Ettiègne-Traoré, V.; Satten, G.A.; Anoma, C.K.; Maurice, C.; Kadjo, J.C.; Coulibaly, I.M.; Wiktor, S.Z.; Greenberg, A.E.; et al. Effect of interventions to control sexually transmitted disease on the incidence of HIV infection in female sex workers. *AIDS* **2001**, *15*, 1421–1431. [CrossRef]
8. Olsen, G.A. Consumption of antibiotics in Greenland, 1964–1970. IV. Changes in the sensitivity of N. gonorrhoeae to antibiotics. *Br. J. Vener. Dis.* **1973**, *49*, 33–41. [CrossRef]
9. Kenyon, C.; Laumen, J.; Van Dijck, C. Could intensive screening for gonorrhoea/chlamydia in PrEP cohorts select for resistance? Historical lessons from a mass treatment campaign in Greenland. *Sex. Transm. Dis.* **2019**. [CrossRef]
10. McNamara, L.A.; MacNeil, J.R.; Cohn, A.C.; Stephens, D.S. Mass chemoprophylaxis for control of outbreaks of meningococcal disease. *Lancet Infect. Dis.* **2018**, *18*, e272–e281. [CrossRef]
11. Stephens, D.S.; Greenwood, B.; Brandtzaeg, P. Epidemic meningitis, meningococcaemia, and Neisseria meningitidis. *Lancet* **2007**, *369*, 2196–2210. [CrossRef]
12. Ala'Aldeen, D.A.; Neal, K.R.; Ait-Tahar, K.; Nguyen-Van-Tam, J.S.; English, A.; Falla, T.J.; Hawkey, P.M.; Slack, R.C. Dynamics of meningococcal long-term carriage among university students and their implications for mass vaccination. *J. Clin. Microbiol.* **2000**, *38*, 2311–2316. [PubMed]
13. Glover, J. The cerebro-spinal fever epidemic of 1917 at X depot. *Epidemiol. Infect.* **1918**, *17*, 350–365. [CrossRef] [PubMed]
14. Rotman, E.; Seifert, H.S. The genetics of Neisseria species. *Annu. Rev. Genet.* **2014**, *48*, 405–431. [CrossRef]
15. Lu, Q.F.; Cao, D.M.; Su, L.L.; Li, S.B.; Ye, G.B.; Zhu, X.Y.; Wang, J. Genus-Wide Comparative Genomics Analysis of Neisseria to Identify New Genes Associated with Pathogenicity and Niche Adaptation of Neisseria Pathogens. *Int. J. Genomics* **2019**, *2019*, 6015730. [CrossRef] [PubMed]
16. Tsoumanis, A.; Hens, N.; Kenyon, C.R. Is screening for chlamydia and gonorrhea in men who have sex with men associated with reduction of the prevalence of these infections? a systematic review of observational studies. *Sex. Transm. Dis.* **2018**, *45*, 615–622. [CrossRef] [PubMed]
17. Ghani, A.C.; Swinton, J.; Garnett, G.P. The role of sexual partnership networks in the epidemiology of gonorrhea. *Sex. Transm. Dis.* **1997**, *24*, 45–56. [CrossRef]
18. Garnett, G.P.; Mertz, K.J.; Finelli, L.; Levine, W.C.; St Louis, M.E. The transmission dynamics of gonorrhoea: Modelling the reported behaviour of infected patients from Newark, New Jersey. *Philos. Trans. R. Soc. Lond. B Biol. Sci.* **1999**, *354*, 787–797. [CrossRef]

19. Kenyon, C.; Delva, W. It's the network, stupid: A population's sexual network connectivity determines its STI prevalence. *F1000Res.* **2018**, *7*, 1880. [CrossRef]
20. Buyze, J.; Vandenberghe, W.; Hens, N.; Kenyon, C. Current levels of gonorrhoea screening in MSM in Belgium may have little effect on prevalence: A modelling study. *Epidemiol. Infect.* **2018**, *146*, 333–338. [CrossRef]
21. Chen, M.; Zhang, C.; Zhang, X.; Chen, M. Meningococcal quinolone resistance originated from several commensal Neisseria species. *Antimicrob.Agents Chemother.* **2019**, *64*, e01494-19. [CrossRef]
22. Bowler, L.D.; Zhang, Q.Y.; Riou, J.Y.; Spratt, B.G. Interspecies recombination between the penA genes of Neisseria meningitidis and commensal Neisseria species during the emergence of penicillin resistance in N. meningitidis: Natural events and laboratory simulation. *J. Bacteriol.* **1994**, *176*, 333–337. [CrossRef] [PubMed]
23. Wadsworth, C.B.; Arnold, B.J.; Sater, M.R.A.; Grad, Y.H. Azithromycin Resistance through Interspecific Acquisition of an Epistasis-Dependent Efflux Pump Component and Transcriptional Regulator in Neisseria gonorrhoeae. *mBio* **2018**, *9*, e01419-18. [CrossRef] [PubMed]
24. Bash, M.C.; Matthias, K.A. Antibiotic Resistance in Neisseria. *Antimicrob. Drug Res.* **2017**, *2*, 843.
25. Saez-Nieto, J.A.; Perucha, M.; Casamayor, H.; Marcen, J.J.; Llacer, A.; Garcia-Barreno, B.; Casal, J. Outbreak of infection caused by Neisseria meningitidis group C type 2 in a nursery. *J. Infect.* **1984**, *8*, 49–55. [CrossRef]
26. Block, C.; Raz, R.; Frasch, C.E.; Ephros, M.; Greif, Z.; Talmon, Y.; Rosin, D.; Bogokowsky, B. Re-emergence of meningococcal carriage on three-year follow-up of a kibbutz population after whole-community chemoprophylaxis. *Eur. J. Clin. Microbiol. Infect. Dis.* **1993**, *12*, 505–511. [CrossRef]
27. Jackson, L.A.; Alexander, E.R.; Debolt, C.A.; Swenson, P.D.; Boase, J.; McDowell, M.G.; Reeves, M.W.; Wenger, J.D. Evaluation of the use of mass chemoprophylaxis during a school outbreak of enzyme type 5 serogroup B meningococcal disease. *Pediatr. Infect. Dis. J.* **1996**, *15*, 992–998. [CrossRef]
28. Pearce, M.C.; Sheridan, J.W.; Jones, D.M.; Lawrence, G.W.; Murphy, D.M.; Masutti, B.; McCosker, C.; Douglas, V.; George, D.; O'Keefe, A.; et al. Control of group C meningococcal disease in Australian aboriginal children by mass rifampicin chemoprophylaxis and vaccination. *Lancet* **1995**, *346*, 20–23. [CrossRef]
29. Millar, J.W.; Siess, E.E.; Feldman, H.A.; Silverman, C.; Frank, P. In vivo and in vitro resistance to sulfadiazine in strains of Neisseria meningitidis. *JAMA* **1963**, *186*, 139–141. [CrossRef]
30. Neal, K.; Irwin, D.; Davies, S.; Kaczmarski, E.; Wale, M. Sustained reduction in the carriage of Neisseria meningitidis as a result of a community meningococcal disease control programme. *Epidemiol. Infect.* **1998**, *121*, 487–493. [CrossRef] [PubMed]
31. Zalmanovici Trestioreanu, A.; Fraser, A.; Gafter-Gvili, A.; Paul, M.; Leibovici, L. Antibiotics for preventing meningococcal infections. *Cochrane Database Syst. Rev.* **2011**, CD004785. [CrossRef] [PubMed]
32. Stephens, D. Neisseria meningitidis. In *Mandell, Douglas, and Bennett's Principles and Practice of Infectious Diseases*; Bennett, J.E., Dolin, R., Blaser, M.J., Eds.; Elsevier Health Sciences: Amsterdam, The Netherlands, 2019.
33. Unemo, M.; Shafer, W.M. Antimicrobial resistance in Neisseria gonorrhoeae in the 21st century: Past, evolution, and future. *Clin. Microbiol. Rev.* **2014**, *27*, 587–613. [CrossRef] [PubMed]
34. Ito, M.; Deguchi, T.; Mizutani, K.S.; Yasuda, M.; Yokoi, S.; Ito, S.; Takahashi, Y.; Ishihara, S.; Kawamura, Y.; Ezaki, T. Emergence and spread of Neisseria gonorrhoeae clinical isolates harboring mosaic-like structure of penicillin-binding protein 2 in Central Japan. *Antimicrob. Agents Chemother.* **2005**, *49*, 137–143. [CrossRef] [PubMed]
35. Tanaka, M.; Nakayama, H.; Huruya, K.; Konomi, I.; Irie, S.; Kanayama, A.; Saika, T.; Kobayashi, I. Analysis of mutations within multiple genes associated with resistance in a clinical isolate of Neisseria gonorrhoeae with reduced ceftriaxone susceptibility that shows a multidrug-resistant phenotype. *Int J Antimicrob Agents* **2006**, *27*, 20–26. [CrossRef] [PubMed]
36. Furuya, R.; Onoye, Y.; Kanayama, A.; Saika, T.; Iyoda, T.; Tatewaki, M.; Matsuzaki, K.; Kobayashi, I.; Tanaka, M. Antimicrobial resistance in clinical isolates of Neisseria subflava from the oral cavities of a Japanese population. *J. Infect. Chemother.* **2007**, *13*, 302–304. [CrossRef]
37. Kenyon, C.; Buyze, J.; Wi, T. Antimicrobial consumption and susceptibility of Neisseria gonorrhoeae: A global ecological analysis. *Front. Med.* **2018**, *5*, 329. [CrossRef]
38. Dong, H.V.; Pham, L.Q.; Nguyen, H.T.; Nguyen, M.X.B.; Nguyen, T.V.; May, F.; Le, G.M.; Klausner, J.D. Decreased Cephalosporin Susceptibility of Oropharyngeal Neisseria Species in Antibiotic-Using Men-who-have-sex-with-men of Hanoi, Vietnam. *Clin. Infect. Dis.* **2019**, ciz365. [CrossRef]

39. Bolan, R.K.; Beymer, M.R.; Weiss, R.E.; Flynn, R.P.; Leibowitz, A.A.; Klausner, J.D. Doxycycline Prophylaxis to Reduce Incident Syphilis among HIV-Infected Men Who Have Sex With Men Who Continue to Engage in High-Risk Sex: A Randomized, Controlled Pilot Study. *Sex. Transm. Dis.* **2015**, *42*, 98–103. [CrossRef]
40. Molina, J.M.; Charreau, I.; Chidiac, C.; Pialoux, G.; Cua, E.; Delaugerre, C.; Capitant, C.; Rojas-Castro, D.; Fonsart, J.; Bercot, B.; et al. Post-exposure prophylaxis with doxycycline to prevent sexually transmitted infections in men who have sex with men: An open-label randomised substudy of the ANRS IPERGAY trial. *Lancet Infect. Dis.* **2017**, *18*, 308–317. [CrossRef]
41. Knapp, J.S. Historical perspectives and identification of Neisseria and related species. *Clin Microbiol Rev.* **1988**, *1*, 415–431. [CrossRef]
42. Kenyon, C. How actively should we screen for chlamydia and gonorrhoea in MSM and other high-ST-prevalence populations as we enter the era of increasingly untreatable infections? A viewpoint. *J. Med. Microbiol.* **2018**, *68*, 132–135. [CrossRef]
43. Kenyon, C.; Schwartz, I.S. A combination of high sexual network connectivity and excess antimicrobial usage induce the emergence of antimicrobial resistance in Neisseria gonorrhoeae. *Emerg. Infect. Dis.* **2018**, *24*, 1195–1203. [CrossRef] [PubMed]
44. Dretler, A.W.; Rouphael, N.G.; Stephens, D.S. Progress toward the global control of Neisseria meningitidis: 21st century vaccines, current guidelines, and challenges for future vaccine development. *Hum. Vaccin. Immunother.* **2018**, *14*, 1146–1160. [CrossRef] [PubMed]
45. Marshall, H.S.; McMillan, M.; Koehler, A.P.; Lawrence, A.; Sullivan, T.R.; MacLennan, J.M.; Maiden, M.C.J.; Ladhan, S.N.; Ramsay, M.E.; Trotter, C.; et al. Meningococcal B Vaccine and Meningococcal Carriage in Adolescents in Australia. *N. Engl. J. Med.* **2020**, *382*, 318–327. [CrossRef] [PubMed]
46. Marshall, H.S.; McMillan, M.; Koehler, A.; Lawrence, A.; MacLennan, J.; Maiden, M.; Ramsay, M.; Ladhani, S.N.; Trotter, C.; Borrow, R.; et al. B Part of It School Leaver protocol: An observational repeat cross-sectional study to assess the impact of a meningococcal serogroup B (4CMenB) vaccine programme on carriage of Neisseria meningitidis. *BMJ Open* **2019**, *9*, e027233. [CrossRef] [PubMed]
47. Terranova, L.; Principi, N.; Bianchini, S.; Di Pietro, G.; Umbrello, G.; Madini, B.; Esposito, S. Neisseria meningitidis serogroup B carriage by adolescents and young adults living in Milan, Italy: Prevalence of strains potentially covered by the presently available meningococcal B vaccines. *Hum. Vaccin. Immunother.* **2018**, *14*, 1070–1074. [CrossRef]
48. Balmer, P.; Burman, C.; Serra, L.; York, L.J. Impact of meningococcal vaccination on carriage and disease transmission: A review of the literature. *Hum. Vaccin. Immunother.* **2018**, *14*, 1118–1130. [CrossRef]
49. Gianchecchi, E.; Piccini, G.; Torelli, A.; Rappuoli, R.; Montomoli, E. An unwanted guest: Neisseria meningitidis—Carriage, risk for invasive disease and the impact of vaccination with insight on Italy incidence. *Expert Rev. Anti. Infect. Ther.* **2017**, *15*, 689–701. [CrossRef]
50. Kenyon, C. Comment on "Effectiveness of a Group B outer membrane vesicle meningococcal vaccine in preventing hospitalization from gonorrhea in New Zealand: A retrospective cohort study. *Vaccines* 2019, *1*, 5, doi:10.3390/vaccines7010005". *Vaccines* **2019**, *7*, 31. [CrossRef]
51. Paynter, J.; Goodyear-Smith, F.; Morgan, J.; Saxton, P.; Black, S.; Petousis-Harris, H.J.V. Effectiveness of a Group B Outer Membrane Vesicle Meningococcal Vaccine in Preventing Hospitalization from Gonorrhea in New Zealand: A Retrospective Cohort Study. *Vaccines* **2019**, *7*, 5. [CrossRef]
52. Petousis-Harris, H.; Paynter, J.; Morgan, J.; Saxton, P.; McArdle, B.; Goodyear-Smith, F.; Black, S. Effectiveness of a group B outer membrane vesicle meningococcal vaccine against gonorrhoea in New Zealand: A retrospective case-control study. *Lancet* **2017**, *390*, 1603–1610. [CrossRef]

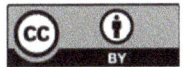

© 2020 by the author. Licensee MDPI, Basel, Switzerland. This article is an open access article distributed under the terms and conditions of the Creative Commons Attribution (CC BY) license (http://creativecommons.org/licenses/by/4.0/).

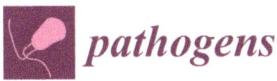

Review

The Laboratory Diagnosis of *Neisseria gonorrhoeae*: Current Testing and Future Demands

Thomas Meyer [1,*] and Susanne Buder [2]

1. Department of Dermatology, Venerology and Allergology, St. Josef Hospital, Ruhr-University, 44791 Bochum, Germany
2. German Consiliary Laboratory for Gonococci, Department of Dermatology and Venerology, Vivantes Hospital Berlin, 12351 Berlin, Germany; susanne.buder@vivantes.de
* Correspondence: t.meyer@klinikum-bochum.de; Tel.: +49-234-509-6014

Received: 7 January 2020; Accepted: 29 January 2020; Published: 31 January 2020

Abstract: The ideal laboratory test to detect *Neisseria gonorrhoeae* (*Ng*) should be sensitive, specific, easy to use, rapid, and affordable and should provide information about susceptibility to antimicrobial drugs. Currently, such a test is not available and presumably will not be in the near future. Thus, diagnosis of gonococcal infections presently includes application of different techniques to address these requirements. Microscopy may produce rapid results but lacks sensitivity in many cases (except symptomatic urogenital infections in males). Highest sensitivity to detect *Ng* was shown for nucleic acid amplification technologies (NAATs), which, however, are less specific than culture. In addition, comprehensive analysis of antibiotic resistance is accomplished only by in vitro antimicrobial susceptibility testing of cultured isolates. As a light at the end of the tunnel, new developments of molecular techniques and microfluidic systems represent promising opportunities to design point-of-care tests for rapid detection of *Ng* with high sensitivity and specificity, and there is reason to hope that such tests may also provide antimicrobial resistance data in the future.

Keywords: gonorrhea; diagnostic; microscopy; culture; antimicrobial resistance; NAAT; point-of-care test; microfluidic

---

1. Introduction

Neisseria gonorrhoeae (*Ng*) infections belong to the most frequent sexually transmitted infections with worldwide around 87 million new infections per year according to WHO estimations [1]. Of these, about 4 million occur in Europe, North America, Australia, and New Zeeland. The vast majority (>80 million) of gonococcal infections are in low- and middle-income countries of Asia, Africa, Latin America, and the Caribbean [1], but increasing incidence is reported in Europe and the USA [2,3]. In Europe, men having sex with men (MSM) accounted for almost half of the reported cases [3]. Transmission of the bacteria is by direct mucosal contact and may lead to infections at the urethra, endocervix, rectum, pharynx, or conjunctiva. While 90% of male urethral infections present with discharge or dysuria, less than 50% of female urethral and cervical infections are symptomatic, and most rectal infections and almost all pharyngeal infections are asymptomatic [4–6]. By transluminal dissemination, starting from the urethral or endocervical mucosa, *Ng* may cause ascending infections resulting in epididymo-orchitis, salpingitis, and pelvic inflammatory disease (PID) [7–9]. In rare cases, the bacteria may spread systemically resulting in severe complications like fever/septicemia, arthritis, tenosynovitis, endocarditis, or vasculitis [10]. In addition, gonococcal infection in pregnancy is associated with adverse pregnancy outcomes, like low birth weight infants, small for gestational age infants, and transmission to newborns that may result in conjunctivitis (ophthalmia neonatorum) and oropharyngeal infections [11,12].

Due to the variety of symptoms that are largely not specific for gonorrhea, timely and accurate laboratory testing of symptomatic patients is required including resistance testing of *Ng*-positive cases for targeted antimicrobial treatment. In addition, screening of key populations to identify and treat asymptomatic infections is no less important to reduce transmission of infection and to control spreading of antibiotic resistance. Hence, the following conditions indicate laboratory testing of gonococcal infection: diagnostic evaluation of clinical symptoms, treatment monitoring, sexual partner(s) diagnosed with *Ng*, other diagnosed STI, new sexual partners or frequently changed sexual partners, and sexual abuse. In the absence of laboratory diagnostics in resource-poor settings, *Ng* infection is usually identified by clinical manifestations combined with medical history and a typical incubation period (2–8 days). However, even classical clinical symptoms like male purulent discharge and urethritis or purulent vaginal discharge or proctitis are not sufficient evidence of gonorrhea, as various other pathogens can cause very similar or identical images. The syndromic approach may possibly suffice for urethral discharge in men but has poor sensitivity and specificity to detect infections in women and non-urethral infection in men, potentially resulting in inadequate treatment with the risk of inducing resistance. It is therefore essential to make laboratory testing available to resource-limited settings.

Laboratory diagnosis of gonococcal infection is established by direct detection of the pathogen in urogenital, anorectal, pharyngeal, or conjunctival swab specimens or first-catch urine. Presently, several different techniques are available for *Ng* detection, of which culture and nucleic acid amplification technologies (NAATs) are best suited [13]. Microscopy of stained urogenital specimens can also be used in certain cases. DNA probe assays, antigen tests, and serology to detect antibodies against *Ng* are not recommended for laboratory testing due to insufficient sensitivity and specificity [13].

During the last decades, diagnostic procedures have been improved continuously, resulting in a better management of individual patients. There are, however, some public health issues to be considered in this context.

1. Improvements of *Ng* testing resulted in increased detection rates that may have influenced epidemiologic data (i.e., higher detection rates do not necessarily indicate an increase in transmitted infections but may just reflect more sensitive and more frequent testing). For instance, introduction of NAATs in routine diagnostic testing have shown pharyngeal and rectal infection to be much more prevalent than previously assumed [14].
2. Since rectal and pharyngeal infections, as well as cervical infections in women, are frequently asymptomatic and will be missed by symptom-based examinations, laboratory testing should consider inclusion of both urogenital, anorectal, and pharyngeal samples, depending on sexual behavior, to identify infected individuals with higher sensitivity [5,15,16].
3. NAAT-based treatment monitoring has improved identification of treatment failures that particularly relate to pharyngeal infections [17]. Considering the presence of non-gonococcal *Neisseria* species at the pharyngeal mucosa that may transfer resistance to *Ng* [18,19], the pharynx has been suggested an important site for resistance development. Currently, the frequency and impact of genetic exchange in the pharynx is not known exactly but is important to be clarified, as it would strongly support pharyngeal screening and clearance of pharyngeal infections to be essential.

The objective of this review article is to summarize current diagnostic procedures for *Ng* detection according to recommendations of several guidelines and to review recent advances and novel developments that may potentially improve *Ng* diagnostic testing, based on publications primarily of the last 5 years identified by a PubMed literature search.

2. Microscopy

Direct microscopy is suitable in defined settings for the detection of Ng as a point-of-care test. Depending on the clinical picture, direct microscopy may be a valid diagnostic tool in settings with more modest resources.

For direct microscopy, two different staining methods are used: methylene blue staining and Gram´s staining. To prepare a staining preparation, the secretion is spread out in a thin layer on a microscope slide and is heated for fixation. For methylene blue staining, the slide is coated with 1% aqueous methylene blue solution or immersed in a cuvette. After a short exposure (15 s), the preparation is rinsed with water and dried between groundwood filter paper. At methylene blue staining, all bacteria turn blue. It should only be used as a diagnostic criterion for uncomplicated male urethritis in combination with typical clinical symptoms. In women's gonorrhea and all other manifestations of disease, Gram´s staining is required [20,21]. Complete staining sets are commercially available. It allows the differentiation into Gram-negative (red) and Gram-positive (blue-violet) bacteria following a stepwise procedure of staining.

At high magnification (1000×), the leukocyte-rich sites are searched and examined with oil immersion. The typical pattern for gonococci is the paired (diplococci), piled, intraleukocytic storage. Diplococci are perpendicular to each other, have the same size and bean or kidney shape. In Gram´s staining, Ng shows as Gram-negative diplococci, often intracellular in polymorphonuclear leukocytes with typical morphology (Figure 1). However, detection of extracellular diplococci, especially in connection with a typical clinical picture, also indicates the presence of Ng. The detection is doubtful if atypical Gram-negative or Gram-labile diplococci are present. In symptomatic male urethritis, the sensitivity of Gram´s staining is up to 95% and highly specific (97%) for an experienced examiner. In endocervical samples, the sensitivity decreases to 40–60% [21,22]. In asymptomatic patients and in pharyngeal and rectal smears, the sensitivity is extremely low, and the method is not recommended [23]. Other bacteria, especially other *Neisseria* species, which have a similar morphology, compromise the microscopic result in extragenital specimens. In asymptomatic patients, the load of gonococci to be detected is usually too low.

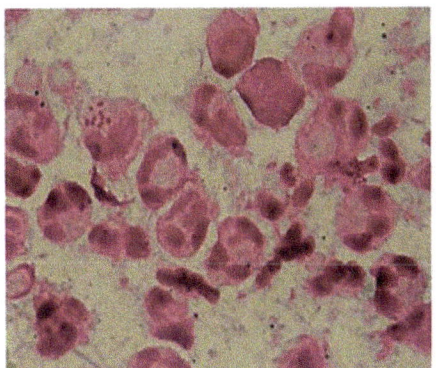 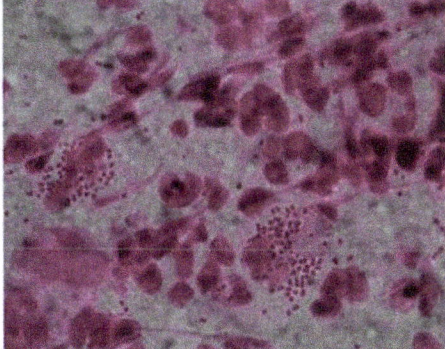

Figure 1. Gram stain from a male urethral swab, depiction of polymorphonuclear leukocytes (PMNL) with Gram-negative intracellular diplococci. The left and right picture represent two different microscopic slides prepared from the same swab.

3. Culture

Antimicrobial resistance in Ng is a severe problem worldwide, and reliable results are indispensable preconditions for a successful therapy. Bacterial culture is sensitive and highly specific. In urogenital specimens, sensitivity may reach 85–95% under optimal conditions [23,24], and specificity is up to

100% when species identification is performed, as shown below. Up to now, it is the only method which allows complete antimicrobial susceptibility testing.

As an example, culture of *Ng* from a male urethral swab is shown in Figure 2. Cultivation does not succeed equally well from every sample material. Smear materials from the urethra and cervix are favorable. Bacterial culture from conjunctival, rectal, and oropharyngeal samples require optimal growth conditions, are time consuming, and often frustrating, especially in the case of throat swabs. Vaginal swab specimens and urine are rarely successfully cultivated [23,25,26].

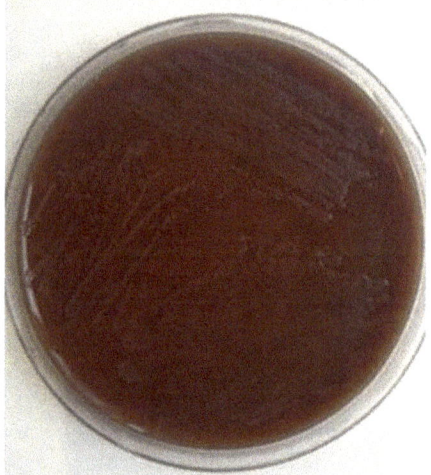

Figure 2. Culture of *Neisseria gonorrhoeae* (*Ng*) from a male urethral swab.

Gonococci are very demanding and fastidious pathogens. They do not tolerate dehydration and should be inoculated immediately after swab collection onto culture media (nutritious selective culture medium and non-selective culture medium) [27]. Culture plates must be incubated at 35–37 °C and high humidity (70–80%), pH 6.75–7.5, and in a 4–6% CO_2-enriched atmosphere. After 18–24 (–48) h, small, shiny gray colonies appear, whereby colony growth variations are possible [23]. After cultivation, identification of *Ng* is assessed by combining several detection methods. A presumptive identification is performed by microscopic Gram´s staining preparation and positive cytochrome oxidase reaction. To confirm the identification and distinguish between other *Neisseria* species like *Neisseria meningitidis* and apathogenic *Neisseria* spp. especially in extragenital sites, biochemical tests, immunological test, spectrometric test, or molecular test are applied. In biochemical identification tests (e.g., API-NH, bioMerieux), various enzymatic reactions and metabolic reactions are displayed by color change. The determined numerical profile allows the identification of the pathogen [28]. Alternative coagglutination tests with gonococcal-specific monoclonal antibodies (e.g., Phadebact Monoclonal GC test, MKL diagnostics; Gonocheck II TCS Biosciences Ltd.) can be performed [28,29].

Furthermore, mass spectrometric identification of *Ng* as a culture-based detection method can be used. MALDI-TOF (matrix-assisted laser desorption ionization time-of-flight) mass spectrometry identifies bacteria that can be taken directly from the agar plate. The result is a spectral fingerprint that can be assigned to the respective microorganism. The method has become established for the detection of *Ng* [30], with a reported positive predictive value of 99.3% [31,32]. However, results should be interpreted with caution for *Ng* and commensal *Neisseria* species when isolated from extragenital and oropharyngeal samples [33]. Molecular confirmation of *Ng* can also be performed using NAATs (see Section 5). Gonococcal typing and genome sequencing are mostly reserved for scientific, epidemiological, and forensic questions.

4. Antimicrobial Susceptibility Testing

Antimicrobial susceptibility testing is one of the most important procedures while processing *Ng*. This allows a reliable statement about the possible effectiveness of an antimicrobial therapeutic agent. Usually, the testing is performed as an indication of the minimum inhibitory concentration (MIC) of an antimicrobial agent in μg/ml or mg/l that inhibits growth. Various breakpoint standards are available for the assessment of susceptibility. It should therefore always be clear according to which standard the assessment is made. Currently, the following two standards are mainly used: CLSI (Clinical and Laboratory Standards Institute) (https://clsi.org/) or EUCAST (European Committee for Antimicrobial Susceptibility Testing) (http://www.eucast.org/clinical_breakpoints/). In addition, national antibiotic sensitivity test committees exist and should be consulted. MIC breakpoints were divided into three categories: "susceptible", "intermediate", and "resistant". Since 2019, EUCAST has been introducing a new classification split into "susceptible", "susceptible with increased exposure", and "resistant". In comparison, the breakpoints for *Ng* of the annually revised and freely accessible recommendations of EUCAST are slightly lower than the ones recommended by CLSI. EUCAST provides no information to zone diameter breakpoints and hence no information on disc diffusion testing. Currently, the main difference for *Ng* breakpoints between the two standards exists for azithromycin. CLSI provides no breakpoints for azithromycin. EUCAST changed from defined breakpoints to an epidemiological cut-off (ECOFF) in 2019. The ECOFF of 1 mg/L applies now to report acquired resistance.

Before performing susceptibility testing, it is important to select a test panel that is appropriate for the pathogen, the expected resistance, and the possible therapy options. There are three main test options for determining susceptibility: agar dilution method, MIC gradient strip test method, and disc diffusions assay. Regardless of the test method, strict and constant quality assurance, the use of WHO control strains, and intra-laboratory and external quality control assessments are required [34,35].

A limited qualitative estimation of antimicrobial susceptibility can be obtained by using a disc diffusion assay [36]. Thereby, discs containing defined antibiotic concentrations are placed on the agar surface. The antibiotic agent diffuses into the culture medium and inhibits growth. After incubation, the inhibition zone diameters are measured in mm. The growth inhibition zone is considered an approximation of the susceptibility (Figure 3). Several disc diffusion methods are described, and the method is only recommended when MIC determination cannot be performed, e.g., due to limited resources [37–39]. Therapeutically relevant disc diffusion results should be supplemented by confirmation tests using other methods.

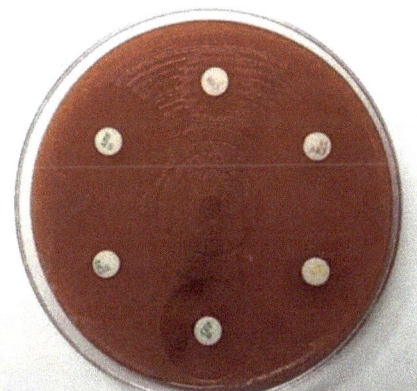

Figure 3. Disc diffusion assay (exemplary, no presentation of *Ng* testing). Photo by Andreas Gross (MVZ Laboratory Krone GbR, Bad Salzuflen, Germany).

The agar dilution method is the WHO-recommended gold standard method for antimicrobial susceptibility testing in *Ng*. A defined series of concentrations of an antibiotic substance is incorporated into nutrient medium. The corresponding growth inhibition is read off in relation to the rising concentration of the antibiotic. The lowest concentration that inhibits growth gives the MIC value in µg/ml (mg/l). However, this method is complex and predominantly suitable for a large number of tests [23]. A similar approach with broth microdilution has been developed but not established as a standard testing method so far [40].

Therefore, the standardized and quality-assured MIC gradient stripe test method (Etest), which correlates with the agar dilution method, is currently the preferred method [23,41,42]. MIC gradient stripe tests are plastic test strips with a predefined concentration gradient for a single antibiotic (Figure 4). The antibiotic agent diffuses into the culture medium, and the elliptical growth inhibition can be read off after incubation by using the printed MIC scale in µg/mL (mg/L). In 2018, various manufacturers of MIC strip test (MIC Test Strips—Liofilchem, M.I.C.Evaluator—Oxoid, and Ezy MIC Strip—HiMedia) were compared and evaluated compared to the reference Etest by bioMérieux for Ng testing. None of the tests met the high standards of Etest. M.I.C.Evaluator strips did not offer the antibiotic panel relevant for Ng testing. Ezy MIC strips showed inconsistent accuracy and quality. Liofilchem MIC Test Strips proofed relatively accurately but were still not fully comparable to Etest (bioMerieux) results [42,43]. In particular, testing of azithomycin is difficult, and test results can vary considerably [44].

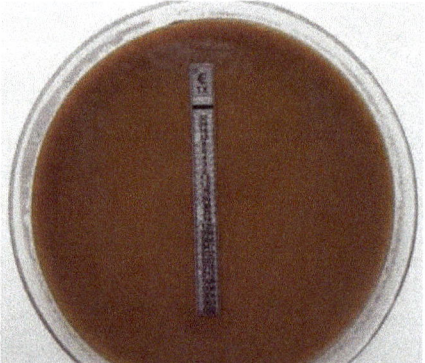

Figure 4. Minimum inhibitory concentration (MIC) gradient strip test method.

Some Ng strains carry a plasmid that encodes a high-level resistance to penicillin. This can be rapidly detected by color change using the Nitrocefin test. However, a negative ß-lactamase test does not exclude low-level penicillin resistance [45].

Recent studies show that early transcriptional changes upon exposure to antibiotics may be used to assess antimicrobial resistance (AMR). For Ng, transcripts have been identified that are differentially regulated in strains susceptible or resistant to ceftriaxone, azithromycin, or ciprofloxacin [46–48]. Quantification of these antibiotic-responsive transcripts results in a signature indicating susceptibility or resistance that may be used as a diagnostic tool in the future. In contrast to DNA-based resistance, test levels of antibiotic-responsive transcripts are independent of genetic mechanisms of resistance, but variance of gene expression may also result from genetic distance effects. Expression levels of porB and rpmB transcripts have been described to diagnose ciprofloxacin resistance in Ng isolates [46], but when testing a genetically more diverse panel of isolates' expression levels of the two markers, they were no longer able to differentiate between susceptible and resistant strains [47]. The technique has great diagnostic potential, but large numbers of diverse Ng isolates from all over the world need to be tested to confirm that specific transcript levels indicate susceptibility or resistance to specific drugs.

5. NAATs

NAATs are the most sensitive techniques to detect *Ng*. Sensitivity and specificity of *Ng* NAATs is generally >95% and >99% in swabs and male first-catch urine (FCU) [4,13]. Currently available commercial tests are based on polymerase chain reaction (PCR) or isothermal transcription-mediated amplification. A list of FDA-approved commercial NAATs as of December 2019 is shown in Table 1. Superiority of NAATs over culture has been demonstrated in a number of studies [13,49–54]. The higher sensitivity of NAAT is partly due to the independence of viable bacteria and applies especially to extragenital specimens [13,14]. Another advantage compared to culture relates to the utility of diverse specimen types that are easier to handle, as no viable bacteria are required [50]. Moreover, NAATs are easier to perform and faster than culture with less hands-on time and the capability of automation allowing high throughput testing [55–57]. In addition, many commercial NAATs were designed to detect both *Ng* and *Chlamydia trachomatis* (*Ct*) in a single reaction [13].

Table 1. Current FDA-approved nucleic acid amplification technologies (NAATs) for detection of *Neisseria gonorrhoeae*.

Assay (Company)	*Ng* Targets	Cleared Specimen Types
Abbott RealTime CT/NG (Abbott)	Opa gene	Women: urine, swabs (vaginal, endocervical) Men: urine, urethral swab
cobas CT/NG (Roche)	Two different targets in the DR 9 region	Women: urine, swabs (vaginal, endocervical) Men: urine
APTIMA Combo 2 Assay (Hologic)	16S-rRNA	urine swabs (vaginal, endocervical, urethral, rectal, pharyngeal)
BD MAX GC BD MAX CT/GC BD MAX CT/GC/TV	OpcA gene	urine (20-60mL of first morning urine recommended), swabs (vaginal endocervical)
BD ProbeTec Neisseria gonorrhoeae (GC) Qx Amplified DNA Assay	Pilin-gene inverting protein homologue	Women: urine, swabs (vaginal, endocervical) Men: urine, urethral swab
BDProbeTec ET Chlamydia trachomatis and Neisseria gonorrhoeae Amplified DNA Assays	Pilin-gene inverting protein homologue	Women: urine, endocervical swab Men: urine, urethral swab
Xpert CT/NG (Cepheid)	Two distinct chromosomal targets	urine swabs (vaginal, endocervical, rectal, pharyngeal)
binx io CT/NG Assay (binx health)	Not specified	vaginal swabs

Notes: As of December 2019.

Although sensitivity of NAATs is superior to other detection methods, it should be considered that diagnostic accuracy may be affected by genetic variations and the genomic plasticity of *Neisseria*. Loss or modification of target regions were shown to reduce sensitivity [58,59], whereas specificity may be diminished by cross-reactive non-pathogenic *Neisseria* species as well as horizontal transfer of *Ng* gene sequences to commensal *Neisseria* [60,61]. Another disadvantage of NAAT-based detection is the lack of information about AMR that still requires isolation of the bacteria by culture and subsequent susceptibility testing. Many commercial NAATs use specific specimen collection kits inappropriate for bacterial culture. However, NAATs may also work properly with nylon flocked swabs in ESwab collection kits [62], from which *Ng* culture succeeded in up to 70% after storage at 4 °C for one day [63], allowing a deferred culture strategy depending on antecedent NAAT results.

To detect male urethral gonococcal infection, first-catch urine (FCU, the first 10–20 mL of micturition) and urethral swabs are equally good, whereas in females, vaginal or endocervical swabs are more sensitive than FCU [13]. FCU is typically self-collected, but vaginal swabs and even meatal swabs may also be collected by the patients themselves and were shown to attain reliable NAAT results [64–66]. Accordingly, guidelines recommend NAAT testing of FCU in men and self-collected vaginal swabs in women, respectively, for laboratory diagnosis of urethral/cervical *Ng* infection [4,13,67].

NAATs are also the most sensitive tests to diagnose extragenital *Ng* infection [14,68,69] and are therefore recommended for laboratory diagnosis of rectal or pharyngeal infection [13,70]. The relevance of testing extragenital sites is mainly based on two findings: (i) additional testing of pharyngeal and rectal swabs was shown to increase the number of infected individuals [5,16]; (ii) patients can be infected at multiple sites [71], and pharyngeal infections are more difficult to treat [72].

Positive NAAT results obtained with extragenital specimens should be confirmed by detection of an alternative target to exclude false positive results due to cross reactivity with commensal *Neisseria* [73]. Confirmatory testing should also be considered in populations with low prevalence (i.e., screening of low-risk populations) with NAAT positive predictive values (PPV) less than 90% [4,74,75]. For routine diagnostic testing, a second test for confirmation seems impractical but may be bypassed using dual target assays including two *Ng* target regions that both need to be amplified for a positive test result [76,77].

Until recently, no NAATs were FDA-cleared for testing extragenital specimens. Thus, compliance with Clinical Laboratory Improvement Amendments (CLIA) for test modifications or equivalent regulatory standards for quality assurance were required. In April 2019, however, two *Ct/Ng* NAATs received FDA approval for testing rectal and pharyngeal specimens (Table 1).

The panel of pathogens included in NAATs for STI testing was recently extended further. Next to *Ct* and *Ng*, *Mycoplsma genitalium* (*Mg*) and *Trichomonas vaginalis* (*Tv*) were incorporated in two commercial assays [57,78]. Performance of BD Max CT/GC/TV assay to detect the three organisms in urine, endocervical, and vaginal swabs from 1990 female and 840 male subjects was consistent with comparator assays for *Ct/Ng* or *Tv* with a sensitivity >95.5% and specificity >98.6% for *Ng* in all specimen types [57]. Similarly, by analyzing 441 urine specimens with the BioRad real-time Dx CT/NG/MG assay, highly concordant results to comparator assays for *Ct/Ng* or *Mg* were described that resulted in a calculated sensitivity and specificity of 92% and 100%, respectively, for *Ng* detection [78].

Some multiplex NAATs allow testing an even more extensive panel of STI pathogens. Selected commercial multiplex NAATs are shown in Table 2. These assays differ with respect to amplification techniques and detection of amplified products, as well as the time to result and the STI panel included. Performance evaluations were published for some of these tests and generally showed good agreement with diagnostic assays for single targets. For instance, the AmpliSense Multiprime FRT real-time PCR assay for *Ct*, *Ng*, *Tv*, and *Mg* was evaluated by comparing it with APTIMA tests for *Ct*, *Ng*, *Tv*, and *Mg* on 209 vaginal swabs and 498 female FCU and 554 male FCU [79]. The authors reported excellent sensitivity and specificity for all pathogens except *Mg*, which lacks sufficient sensitivity. For *Ng*, AmpliSens and APTIMA AC2 results were 100% concordant. The STI FilmArray was applied to 295 clinical specimens and results compared to standard testing [80]. For *Ct* and *Ng*, Roche Amplicor was used as a comparator test and results for *Ct* and *Ng* were 98% and 97% concordant [80]. The STI multiplex assay from Seegene (Anyplex II) uses real-time amplification with multiple primers for seven different STI pathogens. Amplified products were specified by a combination of fluorescence labels and melting point analysis of specially designed oligonucleotides used as hybridization probes. Anyplex II test results largely correspond to results of other diagnostic tests for individual pathogens [81,82]. In a French study, *Ng* test results of 213 specimens obtained with Abbott CT/NG and Anyplex II were 97.2% concordant. Using Abbott CT/NG as a reference test, sensitivity and specificity of Anyplex II were 90% and 98.4%. However, further analysis of samples with discrepant results confirmed one of three Anyplex-positive/Abbott-negative as positive and one of three Anyplex-negative/Abbott-positive test results as negative, indicating sensitivity and specificity of Anyplex II may be even higher [82].

Table 2. Multiplex PCR assays for STI testing.

Assay (Company)	Method of Amplification and Detection	Time to Result	Detected Pathogens
FTD STD 9 (FastTrack Diagnostics)	Real-time PCR Fluorescence	3–4 h	Ct, Ng, Tv, Mg, Uu, Up, Gv, HSV1, HSV2
Anyplex II STI-7 (Seegene)	Real-time PCR fluorescence and melting curve	4–5 h	Ct, Ng, Tv, Mg, Uu, Up, Mh
Amplisense (Interlab Service)	Real-time PCR Fluorescence	3–4 h	Ct, Ng, Tv, Mg
FilmArray STI (BioMerieux)	Nested PCR Fluorescence	1 h	Ct, Ng, Tp, Tv, Mg, HSV1, HSV2, Uu, Hd
Easy Screen (Genetic Signatures)	3-base real-time PCR (Bisufit-PCR) melting curve	3 h	Ct, LGV, Ng, Mg, Tv, Uu, Up, Mh, GBS, Candida, Gv, HSV 1, HSV 2, VZV, Tp
STI Multiplex Aray (Randox Laboratories)	Real-time PCR Fluorescence	30 min	Ct, Ng, Mg, Tv, Uu, Mh, Hd, Tp, HSV 1, HSV 2

Ct: *Chlamydia trachomatis*, Ng: *Neisseria gonorrhoeae*, Tv: *Trichomonas vaginalis*, Mg: *Mycoplasma genitalium*, Uu: *Ureaplasma urealyticum*, Up: *Ureaplasma parvum*, Gv: *Gardnerella vaginalis*, HSV: Herpes simplex virus, Mh: *Mycoplasma hominis*, Hd: *Hemophilus ducreyi*, LGV: Lymphogranuloma venereum, GBS: Group B streptococci, VZV: Varicella zoster virus, Tp: *Treponema pallidum*.

In summary, several studies have shown high clinical sensitivity and specificity of STI multiplex NAATs not inferior to standard NAAT tests for single pathogens or duplex assays. These assays may potentially improve STI diagnostics due the higher content of information. However, depending on the test panel, a controversial discussion about the relevance of test results arose, especially considering microbial agents with low pathogenic potential (like *Ureaplasma parvum* or *Mycoplasma hominis*).

6. Rapid Tests and Point-of-Care Tests (POCT)

Although NAATs are considered the primary tests to detect *Ng*, their use in low- and middle-income countries is greatly limited due to relatively high costs. Management of patients in areas with limited access to laboratory testing is based mainly on clinical symptoms (syndromic-guided management) that, however, may result in inappropriate treatment, potentially increasing the risk of AMR development and spreading. For these regions, low-priced rapid diagnostic tests for *Ng* that can be performed independent from expensive laboratory equipment at the point of care are considered an important approach for confirmation of diagnosis and subsequent targeted treatment. There is also a demand for rapid diagnostic tests in countries with well-developed health care systems. Testing in a central laboratory is associated with increased turnaround times due to sample transport and reporting of test results that requires a follow-up visit of patients in order to start treatment in case of positive test results. Rapid diagnostic tests (RDTs) that can be performed at the point of care may produce test results within a timeframe the patient is willing to wait, allowing initiation of antibiotic treatment and instigation of partner notification at the same visit. Thus, early diagnosis and treatment of *Ng* infection by RDTs may potentially reduce ongoing transmission.

In principle, microscopy can be considered an *Ng* RDT that may be performed at the point of care, given the availability of a microscope. However, microscopic evaluation requires skilled investigators and lacks sensitivity in asymptomatic infections as well as in anorectal and pharyngeal specimens. Due to the presence of non-pathogenic *Neisseria*, specificity is also impaired when analyzing rectal or pharyngeal samples [83].

Other *Ng* RDTs are based on antigen-detection by immunochromatography (lateral flow assays) or optical immunoassays. Several immunochromatographic *Ng* RDTs were evaluated in clinical studies and consistently lack sufficient diagnostic performance with a sensitivity between 12.5% and 94% and a specificity between 89% and 99.8% [84,85]. Sensitivity may be even lower, as some studies used culture or an outdated PCR test with suboptimal sensitivity as the reference method [86–88]. In addition, the PPV of 97% reported in a Japanese study results from analysis of a specimen collection with >50% gonorrhea prevalence that usually does not reflect real situations. In another study, 100% sensitivity and 93% specificity was reported for the Biostar Optical immunoassay; this study, however, included only 5 *Ng*-positive urine specimens [89]. In conclusion, due to insufficient sensitivity and/or specificity, *Ng* RDTs depending on antigen detection are unsuitable to detect *Ng* infection [84].

In contrast, molecular PCR-based rapid tests were shown to have a much better diagnostic performance, comparable to that of reference laboratory NAATs. The GeneXpert CT/NG assay simultaneously detects *Ng* and *Ct* in a closed system and can be used at the point of care. However, the test does not fulfill the classic ASSURED criteria [90] for POCT (i.e., affordable, sensitive, specific, user-friendly, rapid and robust, equipment-free, and deliverable), as it is high-priced, needs electricity, and takes approximately 90 min. Therefore, the GeneXpert assay is usually referred to as a near-patient test rather than a POCT. By analyzing FCU from males, as well as vaginal and cervical swabs, the assay was able to detect *Ng* and *Ct* with high sensitivity (98–100%) and specificity (99.9–100%) that did not differ from reference laboratory NAATs [91]. The significantly higher clinical sensitivity of Xpert results from the low detection limit of 10 *Ng* genome copies [92], which is much lower than for antigen-based assays. The excellent performance was recently confirmed in another evaluation study on vaginal swabs from young South African women [93]. The high specificity results from amplification of two highly specific chromosomal targets that are both required for a positive test result. Therefore, the assay was also evaluated for anorectal and pharyngeal swabs, usually containing numerous commensal Neisseria species. Whereas no significant differences were found by comparing GeneXpert CT/NG with Aptima Combo2 in self-collected rectal swabs [94], sensitivity of GeneXpert was lower when analyzing male pharyngeal samples [95].

Main disadvantages of the GeneXpert system are the relatively high costs and the test duration of about 90 min that may compromise immediate antibiotic treatment in case of positive results if patients are not willing to wait that long and have to return for treatment initiation. Costs of the Xpert assay may vary among high-income countries but will be unacceptably high for resource-poor settings. Some other commercial PCR-based POCTs or near-patient tests to detect *Ng* are now available. Truelab Realtime micro PCR system (Molbio) and Randox STI multiplex array that runs on the Bosch Vivalytic platform are both faster than GeneXpert and take only 50 and 30 min, respectively, but so far, evaluation of both tests has not been published in peer-reviewed papers [96]. The binx io platform (binx health, formerly Atlas Genetics) is based on PCR and electrochemical detection of amplified products. A duplex assay for *Ct* and *Ng* provides results in about 30 min and recently received FDA approval (Table 1). The assay was evaluated in a multicenter study with more than 1500 symptomatic and asymptomatic patients (ClinicalTrials.gov Identifier: NCT03071510). Performance data have not yet been published in a peer-reviewed paper, but according to the company, sensitivity and specificity for *Ng* were 100% and 99.9%, respectively (https://mybinxhealth.com/news/binx-health-receives-fda-510k-clearance-for-rapid-point-of-care-platform-for-womens-health/).

Other NAATs that use isothermal amplification, instead of thermal cycling as in PCR, may reduce both costs and the time to result. Horst et al. recently described a paperfluidic device, integrating swab sample lysis, nucleic acid extraction, DNA amplification by isothermal thermophilic helicase-dependent amplification, and visual detection of amplified products on lateral flow strips. Using this device, *Ng* has been detected with 95% sensitivity and 100% specificity in a proof-of-concept study on 40 urethral and vaginal swab swabs [97]. The turnaround time of this low-cost assay is 80 min and may, according to the authors, be reduced to 60 min, making the assay particularly useful in settings with limited resources. Using recombinase polymerase amplification (RPA) *Ct/Ng* infection can be detected even faster in approximately 15 minutes [98]. A prototype version of this assay (TwistDx RPA assay) runs on the battery-powered Alere i instrument (Alere, Waltham, MA, USA), independent of electricity from the socket. The preliminary evaluation of diagnostic accuracy to detect *Ct* and *Ng* showed sensitivity, specificity, PPV, and NPV > 94% for male FCU, female FCU, and self-collected vaginal swabs [98]. Several other novel developments combining NAAT with microfluidics and nanotechnology that link high sensitivity with rapidity are in the pipeline and represent promising strategies towards a reliable and inexpensive POC testing [96]. These assays are performed on small devices using various microfluidic platforms that direct fluids through channels and reaction chambers for sample preparation and target detection by mechanical and electrokinetic mechanisms. Due to the integration of analytical steps on miniaturized devices, they were also named lab-on-a-chip systems. For example, mCHIP is a portable microfluidic diagnostic device for the detection of antigens and antibodies [99]. It was arranged for diagnosing HIV and syphilis but may also be used for detection of *Ng* and *Ct* antigens. The Vivalytic Analyzer (Bosch) also uses microfluidic techniques for fully automated qualitative and quantitative PCR analysis. The instrument represents an open system able to process diagnostic tests from different manufacturers. Most NAAT-based rapid tests require specific instruments and current supply and are probably unaffordable for low-income countries. However, recently a low-cost, portable analyzer for NAAT-based POCT was described [100] that appears attractive for settings with limited resources.

7. Future Demands

Among the methods for *Ng* detection, NAATs are the most sensitive, but so far, the vast majority of commercially available NAATs does not provide any information about resistance against antimicrobial compounds. Due to the higher sensitivity and easier workflow, as well as more rapid, automated, and high throughput testing, laboratories are increasingly using NAATs instead of culture, leading to a reduction of phenotypic AMR data. In the absence of resistance data, patients were treated empirically, which in the past has led to development of resistance to virtually all antibiotics used for *Ng*, especially in case of monotherapy.

The emergence of AMR strongly impairs the efficacy of *Ng* treatment and represents a significant clinical and public health challenge. Thus, bacterial culture should be attempted whenever possible. When using NAAT as a primary diagnostic test, cultivation of *Ng* subsequent to positive NAAT results frequently fails due to the limited viability of *Ng*. Although deferred culture of the bacteria has been improved using novel flocked swabs for collection of clinical specimens, the probability of successful culture declines with increasing storage time at 4 °C (to 69% after one day and 56% after 2 days) [63], indicating the need of further improvement of specimen collection and culture methods. On the other hand, predictions of AMR might be derived from genotypic data obtained in the context of NAAT analysis, ideally using a rapid molecular POCT.

Molecular alterations causing resistance to antimicrobials used to treat *Ng* were well characterized [101,102], and a number of real-time PCR tests detecting resistance determinants have been published in the last years (see [102] for a review). The assays were designed to detect single resistance mutations or multiple mutations associated with resistance to particular drugs or to a class of antibiotic compounds, like quinolones, macrolides, or beta lactam antibiotics [103–109]. To our knowledge, there is currently only one commercial assay for genotypic resistance testing of *Ng* (SpeeDx ResistancePlus GC for quinolone susceptibility). Some other molecular techniques were published that use a MASSarray iPLEX platform, multiplex bead arrays, and multiplex PCR with high-resolution melting analysis or based on mismatch amplification, allowing a more comprehensive analysis of resistance to multiple antimicrobials [110–113].

Generally, these assays were shown to accurately differentiate between wild type and mutation in both clinical samples and isolated bacteria but differ with respect to performance characteristics. Clinical sensitivity and specificity of some assays is limited, mainly by low *Ng* load and cross-reactive species [102]. Furthermore, prediction of resistance to antimicrobial drugs based on detection of individual resistance determinants is difficult, as development of resistance requires accumulation of several determinants in most cases. In order to standardize interpretation of genetic alterations associated with antibiotic resistance, the Public Health Agency of Canada has developed a web-based system (NG-STAR) for classification of seven genes associated with resistance to three classes of antibiotics (cephalosporins, macrolides, and fluoroquinolones). Currently, prediction of resistance based on genetic changes is most accurate for fluoroquinolones [104,114,115]. The primary mutations associated with ciprofloxacin resistance are located in the quinolone resistance determining region (QRDR) of gyrA, encoding subunit A of DNA gyrase. Additional mutations in parC encoding a subunit of topoisomerase IV are required for high-level resistance [101]. In regions with less prevalent ciprofloxacin resistance (i.e., outside Asia) implementation of genotypic ciprofloxacin resistance testing appears useful, as shown in an American study describing a significant decline of ceftriaxone use when guiding treatment by a PCR-based assay for ciprofloxacin resistance [116].

However, resistance to other antimicrobials used in *Ng* treatment is more complex, as multiple mechanisms contribute to the development of resistance. For instance, resistance to beta lactam antibiotics includes expression of beta lactamases, altered PBPs (point mutation and mosaic variants), increased discharge by efflux pumps, and reduced uptake by porins [102]. Consequently, in these cases, the presence of individual AMR determinants is insufficient to predict phenotypic resistance, but on the other hand, exclusion of any resistance determinant may indicate susceptibility with high probability [104].

In addition to determining the level of resistance analogous to MIC values in bacterial culture, genotypic resistance testing of *Ng* faces several other challenges, like cross-reactivity, especially in extragenital samples [103,106]; mixed infections of susceptible and resistant strains [117]; and the necessity of internal controls to exclude false negative results due to low gonococcal concentrations [118]. In addition, genetic assays are able to detect only known but not new AMR determinants that frequently develop in *Ng*, as we have seen in the past. Thus, any putative commercial genotypic test needs to be modified accordingly in a reasonable period without time-consuming and costly clinical validation.

At present, application of genotypic resistance testing appears to be useful primarily for surveillance of gonococcal resistance. To guide individual therapy of patients, further improvements are required to achieve high diagnostic accuracy and a high predictive value of AMR. This may be achieved in the future by applying whole genome sequencing [47,119,120] and deep learning systems for evaluation of sequencing data that, based on large sets of correlated genotypic and phenotypic data, may provide quantitative information about resistance to particular drugs, similar to the algorithms used in guiding antiretroviral therapy, for instance.

Author Contributions: All authors have read and agree to the published version of the manuscript. S.B. and T.M. both contributed to conceptualization, methodology of literature research, and writing (original draft preparation and review).

Funding: This research received no external funding.

Acknowledgments: We kindly thank Dipl. Biol. Andreas Gross (MVZ Laboratory Krone GbR, Bad Salzuflen, Germany) for the permission to use the image in Figure 1.

Conflicts of Interest: The authors declare no conflict of interest.

References

1. Rowley, J.; Vander Hoorn, S.; Korenromp, E.; Low, N.; Unemo, M.; Abu-Raddad, L.J.; Chico, R. *Chlamydia*, gonorrhoea, trichomoniasis and syphilis: Global prevalence and incidence estimates, 2016. *Bull World Heal. Organ.* **2019**, *97*, 548–562. [CrossRef]
2. European Centre for Disease Prevention and Control. *Gonorrhoea—Annual Epidemiological Report for 2017*; European Centre for Disease Prevention and Control: Stockholm, Sweden, 2019.
3. Department of Health and Human Services. *Sexually Transmitted Disease Surveillance 2018*; Centers for Disease Control and Prevention: Atlanta, GE, USA, 2019. [CrossRef]

4. Fifer, H.; Saunders, J.; Soni, S.; Sadiq, T.; FitzGerald, M. National Guideline for the Management of Infection with *Neisseria gonorrhoeae*. British Association for Sexual Health and HIV Web Site, 2019. Available online: https://www.bashhguidelines.org/media/1208/gc-2019.pdf (accessed on 30 January 2020).
5. Dudareva-Vizule, S.; Haar, K.; Sailer, A.; Wisplinghoff, H.; Wisplinghoff, F.; Marcus, U.; PARIS Study Group. Prevalence of pharyngeal and rectal *Chlamydia trachomatis* and *Neisseria gonorrhoeae* infections among men who have sex with men in Germany. *Sex Transm. Infect.* **2014**, *90*, 46–51. [CrossRef]
6. Buder, S.; Dudareva, S.; Jansen, K.; Loenenbach, A.; Nikisins, S.; Sailer, A.; Guhl, E.; Kohl, P.K.; Bremer, V.; GORENET Study Group. Antimicrobial resistance of *Neisseria gonorrhoeae* in Germany: Low levels of cephalosporin resistance, but high azithromycin resistance. *BMC Infect. Dis.* **2018**, *18*, 44. [CrossRef]
7. McConaghy, J.R.; Panchal, B. Epididymitis: An Overview. *Am. Fam. Physician* **2016**, *94*, 723–726.
8. Reekie, J.; Donovan, B.; Guy, R.; Hocking, J.S.; Kaldor, J.M.; Mak, D.; Preen, D.; Ward, J.; Liu, B. Risk of Pelvic Inflammatory Disease in Relation to *Chlamydia* and Gonorrhea Testing, Repeat Testing, and Positivity: A Population-Based Cohort Study. *Clin. Infect. Dis.* **2018**, *66*, 437–443. [CrossRef]
9. Brunham, R.C.; Gottlieb, S.L.; Paavonen, J. Pelvic inflammatory disease. *N. Engl. J. Med.* **2015**, *372*, 2039–2048. [CrossRef]
10. Belkacem, A.; Caumes, E.; Ouanich, J.; Jarlier, V.; Dellion, S.; Cazenave, B.; Goursaud, R.; Lacassin, F.; Breuil, J.; Patey, O.; et al. Changing patterns of disseminated gonococcal infection in France: Cross-sectional data 2009–2011. *Sex Transm. Infect.* **2013**, *89*, 613–615. [CrossRef]
11. Heumann, C.L.; Quilter, L.A.; Eastment, M.C.; Heffron, R.; Hawes, S.E. Adverse Birth Outcomes and Maternal *Neisseria gonorrhoeae* Infection: A Population-Based Cohort Study in Washington State. *Sex Transm. Dis.* **2017**, *44*, 266–271. [CrossRef]
12. Alexander, E.R. Gonorrhea in the newborn. *Ann. N. Y. Acad. Sci.* **1988**, *549*, 180–186. [CrossRef]
13. Papp, J.R.; Schachter, J.; Gaydos, C.A.; van der Pol, B. Recommendations for the laboratory-based detection of *Chlamydia trachomatis* and *Neisseria gonorrhoeae*—2014. *MMWR Recomm. Rep.* **2014**, *63*, 1–19.
14. Cornelisse, V.J.; Chow, E.P.; Huffam, S.; Fairley, C.K.; Bissessor, M.; De Petra, V.; Howden, B.P.; Denham, I.; Bradshaw, C.S.; Williamson, D.; et al. Increased Detection of Pharyngeal and Rectal Gonorrhea in Men Who Have Sex With Men After Transition From Culture To Nucleic Acid Amplification Testing. *Sex Transm. Dis.* **2017**, *44*, 114–117. [CrossRef]
15. Kent, C.K.; Chaw, J.K.; Wong, W.; Liska, S.; Gibson, S.; Hubbard, G.; Klausner, J.D. Prevalence of rectal, urethral, and pharyngeal *Chlamydia* and gonorrhea detected in 2 clinical settings among men who have sex with men: San Francisco, California, 2003. *Clin. Infect. Dis.* **2005**, *41*, 67–74. [CrossRef]
16. Weston, E.J.; Kirkcaldy, R.D.; Stenger, M.; Llata, E.; Hoots, B.; Torrone, E.A. Narrative Review: Assessment of *Neisseria gonorrhoeae* Infections Among Men Who Have Sex With Men in National and Sentinel Surveillance Systems in the United States. *Sex Transm. Dis.* **2018**, *45*, 243–249. [CrossRef]
17. Allen, V.G.; Mitterni, L.; Seah, C.; Rebbapragada, A.; Martin, I.E.; Lee, C.; Siebert, H.; Towns, L.; Melano, R.G.; Low, D.E. *Neisseria gonorrhoeae* treatment failure and susceptibility to cefixime in Toronto, Canada. *JAMA* **2013**, *309*, 163–170. [CrossRef]
18. Spratt, B.G.; Bowler, L.D.; Zhang, Q.Y.; Zhou, J.; Smith, J.M. Role of interspecies transfer of chromosomal genes in the evolution of penicillin resistance in pathogenic and commensal *Neisseria* species. *J. Mol. Evol.* **1992**, *34*, 115–125. [CrossRef]
19. Wadsworth, C.B.; Arnold, B.J.; Sater, M.R.A.; Grad, Y.H. Azithromycin Resistance through Interspecific Acquisition of an Epistasis-Dependent Efflux Pump Component and Transcriptional Regulator in *Neisseria gonorrhoeae*. *MBio* **2018**, *9*. [CrossRef]
20. Unemo, M.; Seifert, H.S.; Hook, E.W., III; Hawkes, S.; Ndowa, F.; Dillon, J.R. Gonorrhoea. *Nat. Rev. Dis. Primers* **2019**, *5*, 79. [CrossRef]
21. Thorley, N.; Radcliffe, K. The performance and clinical utility of cervical microscopy for the diagnosis of gonorrhoea in women in the era of the NAAT. *Int. J. STD AIDS* **2015**, *26*, 656–660. [CrossRef]
22. Mensforth, S.; Thorley, N.; Radcliffe, K. Auditing the use and assessing the clinical utility of microscopy as a point-of-care test for *Neisseria gonorrhoeae* in a Sexual Health clinic. *Int. J. STD AIDS* **2018**, *29*, 157–163. [CrossRef]

23. Unemo, M.; Ison, C. Gonorrhea. In *Laboratory Diagnosis of Sexually Transmitted Infections, Including Human Immunodeficiency Virus*; Unemo, M., Ballard, R., Ison, C., Lewis, D., Ndowna, F., Peeling, R., Eds.; WHO: Geneva, Switzerland, 2013; Available online: https://www.who.int/reproductivehealth/publications/rtis/9789241505840/en/ (accessed on 30 January 2020).
24. Bignell, C.; Ison, C.A.; Jungmann, E. Gonorrhoea. *Sex Transm. Infect.* **2006**, *82* (Suppl. 4), iv6–iv9. [CrossRef]
25. Ota, K.V.; Tamari, I.E.; Smieja, M.; Jamieson, F.; Jones, K.E.; Towns, L.; Juzkiw, J.; Richardson, S.E. Detection of *Neisseria gonorrhoeae* and *Chlamydia trachomatis* in pharyngeal and rectal specimens using the BD Probetec ET system, the Gen-Probe Aptima Combo 2 assay and culture. *Sex Transm. Infect.* **2009**, *85*, 182–186. [CrossRef]
26. Alexander, S. The challenges of detecting gonorrhoea and *Chlamydia* in rectal and pharyngeal sites: Could we, should we, be doing more? *Sex Transm. Infect.* **2009**, *85*, 159–160. [CrossRef]
27. Visser, M.; van Westreenen, M.; van Bergen, J.; van Benthem, B.H.B. Low gonorrhoea antimicrobial resistance and culture positivity rates in general practice: A pilot study. *Sex Transm. Infect.* **2019**. [CrossRef]
28. Alexander, S.; Ison, C. Evaluation of commercial kits for the identification of *Neisseria gonorrhoeae*. *J. Med. Microbiol.* **2005**, *54*, 827–831. [CrossRef]
29. Dillon, J.R.; Carballo, M.; Pauzé, M. Evaluation of eight methods for identification of pathogenic *Neisseria* species: Neisseria-Kwik, RIM-N, Gonobio-Test, Minitek, Gonochek II, GonoGen, Phadebact Monoclonal GC OMNI Test, and Syva MicroTrak Test. *J. Clin. Microbiol.* **1988**, *26*, 493–497.
30. Carannante, A.; De Carolis, E.; Vacca, P.; Vella, A.; Vocale, C.; De Francesco, M.A.; Cusini, M.; Del Re, S.; Dal Conte, I.; Cristaudo, A.; et al. Evaluation of matrix-assisted laser desorption ionization-time of flight mass spectrometry (MALDI-TOF MS) for identification and clustering of *Neisseria gonorrhoeae*. *BMC Microbiol.* **2015**, *15*, 142. [CrossRef]
31. Buchanan, R.; Ball, D.; Dolphin, H.; Dave, J. Matrix-assisted laser desorption-ionization time-of-flight mass spectrometry for the identification of *Neisseria gonorrhoeae*. *Clin. Microbiol. Infect.* **2016**, *22*, 815. [CrossRef]
32. Schweitzer, V.A.; van Dam, A.P.; Hananta, I.P.; Schuurman, R.; Kusters, J.G.; Rentenaar, R.J. Identification of *Neisseria gonorrhoeae* by the Bruker Biotyper Matrix-Assisted Laser Desorption Ionization-Time of Flight Mass Spectrometry System Is Improved by a Database Extension. *J. Clin. Microbiol.* **2016**, *54*, 1130–1132. [CrossRef]
33. Morel, F.; Jacquier, H.; Desroches, M.; Fihman, V.; Kumanski, S.; Cambau, E.; Decousser, J.W.; Berçot, B. Use of Andromas and Bruker MALDI-TOF MS in the identification of *Neisseria*. *Eur. J. Clin. Microbiol. Infect. Dis.* **2018**, *37*, 2273–2277. [CrossRef]
34. Unemo, M.; Fasth, O.; Fredlund, H.; Limnios, A.; Tapsall, J. Phenotypic and genetic characterization of the 2008 WHO *Neisseria gonorrhoeae* reference strain panel intended for global quality assurance and quality control of gonococcal antimicrobial resistance surveillance for public health purposes. *J. Antimicrob. Chemother.* **2009**, *63*, 1142–1151. [CrossRef]
35. Unemo, M.; Golparian, D.; Sánchez-Busó, L.; Grad, Y.; Jacobsson, S.; Ohnishi, M.; Lahra, M.M.; Limnios, A.; Sikora, A.E.; Wi, T.; et al. The novel 2016 WHO *Neisseria gonorrhoeae* reference strains for global quality assurance of laboratory investigations: Phenotypic, genetic and reference genome characterization. *J. Antimicrob. Chemother.* **2016**, *71*, 3096–3108. [CrossRef]
36. Liu, H.; Taylor, T.H., Jr.; Pettus, K.; Johnson, S.; Papp, J.R.; Trees, D. Comparing the disk-diffusion and agar dilution tests for *Neisseria gonorrhoeae* antimicrobial susceptibility testing. *Antimicrob. Resist. Infect. Control* **2016**, *5*, 46. [CrossRef]
37. Singh, V.; Bala, M.; Kakran, M.; Ramesh, V. Comparative assessment of CDS, CLSI disc diffusion and Etest techniques for antimicrobial susceptibility testing of *Neisseria gonorrhoeae*: A 6-year study. *BMJ Open* **2012**, *2*. [CrossRef]
38. Mal, P.B.; Jabeen, K.; Farooqi, J.; Unemo, M.; Khan, E. Antimicrobial susceptibility testing of *Neisseria gonorrhoeae* isolates in Pakistan by Etest compared to Calibrated Dichotomous Sensitivity and Clinical Laboratory Standards Institute disc diffusion techniques. *BMC Microbiol.* **2016**, *16*, 236. [CrossRef]
39. Enriquez, R.P.; Goire, N.; Kundu, R.; Gatus, B.J.; Lahra, M.M. A comparison of agar dilution with the Calibrated Dichotomous Sensitivity (CDS) and Etest methods for determining the minimum inhibitory concentration of ceftriaxone against *Neisseria gonorrhoeae*. *Diagn. Microbiol. Infect. Dis.* **2016**, *86*, 40–43. [CrossRef]
40. Foerster, S.; Desilvestro, V.; Hathaway, L.J.; Althaus, C.L.; Unemo, M. A new rapid resazurin-based microdilution assay for antimicrobial susceptibility testing of *Neisseria gonorrhoeae*. *J. Antimicrob. Chemother.* **2017**, *72*, 1961–1968. [CrossRef]

41. Liu, H.; Taylor, T.H., Jr.; Pettus, K.; Trees, D. Assessment of Etest as an alternative to agar dilution for antimicrobial susceptibility testing of *Neisseria gonorrhoeae*. *J. Clin. Microbiol.* **2014**, *52*, 1435–1440. [CrossRef]
42. Papp, J.R.; Rowlinson, M.C.; O'Connor, N.P.; Wholehan, J.; Razeq, J.H.; Glennen, A.; Ware, D.; Iwen, P.C.; Lee, L.V.; Hagan, C. Accuracy and reproducibility of the Etest to detect drug-resistant *Neisseria gonorrhoeae* to contemporary treatment. *J. Med. Microbiol.* **2018**, *67*, 68–73. [CrossRef]
43. Jönsson, A.; Jacobsson, S.; Foerster, S.; Cole, M.J.; Unemo, M. Performance characteristics of newer MIC gradient strip tests compared with the Etest for antimicrobial susceptibility testing of *Neisseria gonorrhoeae*. *APMIS* **2018**, *126*, 822–827. [CrossRef]
44. McAuliffe, G.N.; Smith, M.; Cooper, G.; Forster, R.F.; Roberts, S.A. Variability in Azithromycin Susceptibility Results for *Neisseria gonorrhoeae* Obtained Using Gradient MIC Strip and Agar Dilution Techniques. *J. Clin. Microbiol.* **2019**, *57*, e01353–19. [CrossRef]
45. Tapsall, J.W.; Phillips, E.A.; Morris, L.M. Chromosomally mediated intrinsic resistance to penicillin in penicillinase producing strains of *Neisseria gonorrhoeae* isolated in Sydney: Guide to treatment with Augmentin. *Genitourin. Med.* **1987**, *63*, 305–308. [CrossRef]
46. Khazaei, T.; Barlow, J.T.; Schoepp, N.G.; Ismagilov, R.F. RNA markers enable phenotypic test of antibiotic susceptibility in *Neisseria gonorrhoeae* after 10 minutes of ciprofloxacin exposure. *Sci. Rep.* **2018**, *8*, 11606. [CrossRef]
47. Wadsworth, C.B.; Sater, M.R.A.; Bhattacharyya, R.P.; Grad, Y.H. Impact of Species Diversity on the Design of RNA-Based Diagnostics for Antibiotic Resistance in *Neisseria gonorrhoeae*. *Antimicrob. Agents Chemother.* **2019**, *63*. [CrossRef]
48. Zhao, Y.H.; Qin, X.L.; Yang, J.Y.; Liao, Y.W.; Wu, X.Z.; Zheng, H.P. Identification and expression analysis of ceftriaxone resistance-related genes in *Neisseria gonorrhoeae* integrating RNA-Seq data and qRT-PCR validation. *J. Glob. Antimicrob. Resist.* **2019**, *16*, 202–209. [CrossRef]
49. Martin, D.H.; Cammarata, C.; van der Pol, B.; Jones, R.B.; Quinn, T.C.; Gaydos, C.A.; Crotchfelt, K.; Schachter, J.; Moncada, J.; Jungkind, D.; et al. Multicenter evaluation of AMPLICOR and automated cobas AMPLICOR CTT/NG tests for *Neisseria gonorrhoeae*. *J. Clin. Microbiol.* **2000**, *38*, 3544–3549.
50. Cook, R.L.; Hutchison, S.L.; Ostergaard, L.; Braithwaite, R.S.; Ness, R.B. Systematic review: Noninvasive testing for *Chlamydia trachomatis* and *Neisseria gonorrhoeae*. *Ann. Intern. Med.* **2005**, *142*, 914–925. [CrossRef]
51. Van Dyck, E.; Ieven, M.; Pattyn, S.; Van Damme, L.; Laga, M. Detection of *Chlamydia trachomatis* and *Neisseria gonorrhoeae* by enzyme immunoassay, culture, and three nucleic acid amplification tests. *J. Clin. Microbiol.* **2001**, *39*, 1751–1756. [CrossRef]
52. Serra-Pladevall, J.; Caballero, E.; Roig, G.; Juvé, R.; Barbera, M.J.; Andreu, A. Comparison between conventional culture and NAATs for the microbiological diagnosis in gonococcal infection. *Diagn. Microbiol. Infect. Dis.* **2015**, *83*, 341–343. [CrossRef]
53. Bromhead, C.; Miller, A.; Jones, M.; Whiley, D. Comparison of the cobas 4800 CT/NG test with culture for detecting *Neisseria gonorrhoeae* in genital and nongenital specimens in a low-prevalence population in New Zealand. *J. Clin. Microbiol.* **2013**, *51*, 1505–1509. [CrossRef]
54. Van der Pol, B.; Hook, E.W., III; Williams, J.A.; Smith, B.; Taylor, S.N. Performance of the BD CTQx and GCQx Amplified Assays on the BD Viper LT Compared With the BD Viper XTR System. *Sex Transm. Dis.* **2015**, *42*, 521–523. [CrossRef]
55. Cheng, A.; Kirby, J.E. Evaluation of the Hologic gen-probe PANTHER, APTIMA Combo 2 assay in a tertiary care teaching hospital. *Am. J. Clin. Pathol.* **2014**, *141*, 397–403. [CrossRef]
56. Marlowe, E.M.; Hardy, D.; Krevolin, M.; Gohl, P.; Bertram, A.; Arcenas, R.; Seiverth, B.; Schneider, T.; Liesenfeld, O. High-throughput testing of urogenital and extragenital specimens for detection of *Chlamydia trachomatis* and *Neisseria gonorrhoeae* with Cobas CT/NG. *Eur. J. Microbiol. Immunol. Bp.* **2017**, *7*, 176–186. [CrossRef]
57. Van der Pol, B.; Williams, J.A.; Fuller, D.; Taylor, S.N.; Hook, E.W., III. Combined Testing for *Chlamydia*, gonorrhea, and *Trichomonas* by use of the BD Max CT/GC/TV Assay with genitourinary specimen types. *J. Clin. Microbiol.* **2017**, *55*, 155–164. [CrossRef]
58. Whiley, D.M.; Limnios, A.; Moon, N.J.; Gehrig, N.; Goire, N.; Hogan, T.; Lam, A.; Jacob, K.; Lambert, S.B.; Nissen, M.D.; et al. False-negative results using *Neisseria gonorrhoeae* porA pseudogene PCR—A clinical gonococcal isolate with an *N. meningitidis* porA sequence, Australia, March 2011. *Eurosurveillance* **2011**, *16*, 19874.

59. Ison, C.A.; Golparian, D.; Saunders, P.; Chisholm, S.; Unemo, M. Evolution of *Neisseria gonorrhoeae* is a continuing challenge for molecular detection of gonorrhoea: False negative gonococcal porA mutants are spreading internationally. *Sex Transm. Infect.* **2013**, *89*, 197–201. [CrossRef]
60. Upton, A.; Bromhead, C.; Whiley, D.M. *Neisseria gonorrhoeae* false-positive result obtained from a pharyngeal swab by using the Roche cobas 4800 CT/NG assay in New Zealand in 2012. *J. Clin. Microbiol.* **2013**, *51*, 1609–1610. [CrossRef]
61. Frosch, M.; Meyer, T.F. Transformation-mediated exchange of virulence determinants by co-cultivation of pathogenic *Neisseriae*. *FEMS Microbiol. Lett.* **1992**, *100*, 345–349. [CrossRef]
62. Li, J.; Jang, D.; Gilchrist, J.; Smieja, M.; Ewert, R.; MacRitchie, C.; Chernesky, M. Comparison of flocked and aptima swabs and two specimen transport media in the aptima combo 2 assay. *J. Clin. Microbiol.* **2014**, *52*, 3808–3809. [CrossRef]
63. Wind, C.M.; de Vries, H.J.; Schim van der Loeff, M.F.; Unemo, M.; van Dam, A.P. Successful Combination of Nucleic Acid Amplification Test Diagnostics and Targeted Deferred *Neisseria gonorrhoeae* Culture. *J. Clin. Microbiol.* **2015**, *53*, 1884–1990. [CrossRef]
64. Schachter, J.; Chernesky, M.A.; Willis, D.E.; Fine, P.M.; Martin, D.H.; Fuller, D.; Jordan, J.A.; Janda, W.; Hook, E.W., III. Vaginal swabs are the specimens of choice when screening for *Chlamydia trachomatis* and *Neisseria gonorrhoeae*: Results from a multicenter evaluation of the APTIMA assays for both infections. *Sex Transm. Dis.* **2005**, *32*, 725–728. [CrossRef]
65. Stewart, C.M.; Schoeman, S.A.; Booth, R.A.; Smith, S.D.; Wilcox, M.H.; Wilson, J.D. Assessment of self taken swabs versus clinician taken swab cultures for diagnosing gonorrhoea in women: Single centre, diagnostic accuracy study. *BMJ Clin. Res. Ed.* **2012**, *345*, e8107. [CrossRef]
66. Dize, L.; Agreda, P.; Quinn, N.; Barnes, M.R.; Hsieh, Y.H.; Gaydos, C.A. Comparison of self-obtained penile-meatal swabs to urine for the detection of *C. trachomatis*, *N. gonorrhoeae* and *T. vaginalis*. *Sex Transm. Infect.* **2013**, *89*, 305–307. [CrossRef]
67. AWMF. Leitlinie: Sexuell Übertragbare Infektionen (STI)—Beratung, Diagnostik, Therapie, 059-006. 2019. Available online: https://www.awmf.org/uploads/tx_szleitlinien/059-006l_S2k_Sexuell-uebertragbare-Infektionen-Beratung-Diagnostik-Therapie-STI_2019-09.pdf (accessed on 30 January 2020).
68. Page-Shafer, K.; Graves, A.; Kent, C.; Balls, J.E.; Zapitz, V.M.; Klausner, J.D. Increased sensitivity of DNA amplification testing for the detection of pharyngeal gonorrhea in men who have sex with men. *Clin. Infect. Dis.* **2002**, *34*, 173–176. [CrossRef]
69. Schachter, J.; Moncada, J.; Liska, S.; Shayevich, C.; Klausner, J.D. Nucleic acid amplification tests in the diagnosis of chlamydial and gonococcal infections of the oropharynx and rectum in men who have sex with men. *Sex Transm. Dis.* **2008**, *35*, 637–642. [CrossRef]
70. Hughes, G.; Ison, C.; Field, N. *Guidance for the Detection of Gonorrhoea in England*; Public Health England: London, UK, 2014; Available online: https://assets.publishing.service.gov.uk/government/uploads/system/uploads/attachment_data/file/769003/170215_Gonorrhoea_testing_guidance_REVISED__2_.pdf. (accessed on 30 January 2020).
71. Benn, P.D.; Rooney, G.; Carder, C.; Brown, M.; Stevenson, S.R.; Copas, A.; Robinson, A.J.; Ridgway, G.L. *Chlamydia trachomatis* and *Neisseria gonorrhoeae* infection and the sexual behaviour of men who have sex with men. *Sex Transm. Infect.* **2007**, *83*, 106–112. [CrossRef]
72. Fifer, H.; Natarajan, U.; Jones, L.; Alexander, S.; Hughes, G.; Golparian, D.; Unemo, M. Failure of Dual Antimicrobial Therapy in Treatment of Gonorrhea. *N. Engl. J. Med.* **2016**, *374*, 2504–2506. [CrossRef]
73. Palmer, H.M.; Mallinson, H.; Wood, R.L.; Herring, A.J. Evaluation of the specificities of five DNA amplification methods for the detection of *Neisseria gonorrhoeae*. *J. Clin. Microbiol.* **2003**, *41*, 835–837. [CrossRef]
74. Field, N.; Clifton, S.; Alexander, S.; Ison, C.A.; Hughes, G.; Beddows, S.; Tanton, C.; Soldan, K.; Coelho da Silva, F.; Mercer, C.H.; et al. Confirmatory assays are essential when using molecular testing for *Neisseria gonorrhoeae* in low-prevalence settings: Insights from the third National Survey of Sexual Attitudes and Lifestyles (Natsal-3). *Sex Transm. Infect.* **2015**, *91*, 338–341. [CrossRef]
75. Chow, E.P.; Fehler, G.; Read, T.R.; Tabrizi, S.N.; Hocking, J.S.; Denham, I.; Bradshaw, C.S.; Chen, M.Y.; Fairley, C.K. Gonorrhoea notifications and nucleic acid amplification testing in a very low-prevalence Australian female population. *Med. J. Aust.* **2015**, *202*, 321–323. [CrossRef]

76. Tabrizi, S.N.; Unemo, M.; Golparian, D.; Twin, J.; Limnios, A.E.; Lahra, M.; Guy, R.; TTANGO Investigators. Analytical evaluation of GeneXpert CT/NG, the first genetic point-of-care assay for simultaneous detection of *Neisseria gonorrhoeae* and *Chlamydia trachomatis*. *J. Clin. Microbiol.* **2013**, *51*, 1945–1947. [CrossRef]
77. Perry, M.D.; Jones, R.N.; Corden, S.A. Is confirmatory testing of Roche cobas 4800 CT/NG test *Neisseria gonorrhoeae* positive samples required? Comparison of the Roche cobas 4800 CT/NG test with an opa/pap duplex assay for the detection of *N. gonorrhoeae*. *Sex Transm. Infect.* **2014**, *90*, 303–308. [CrossRef]
78. Ursi, D.; Crucitti, T.; Smet, H.; Ieven, M. Evaluation of the Bio-Rad Dx CT/NG/MG®assay for simultaneous detection of *Chlamydia trachomatis*, *Neisseria gonorrhoeae* and *Mycoplasma genitalium* in urine. *Eur. J. Clin. Microbiol. Infect. Dis.* **2016**, *35*, 1159–1163. [CrossRef]
79. Rumyantseva, T.; Golparian, D.; Nilsson, C.S.; Johansson, E.; Falk, M.; Fredlund, H.; Van Dam, A.; Guschin, A.; Unemo, M. Evaluation of the new AmpliSens multiplex real-time PCR assay for simultaneous detection of *Neisseria gonorrhoeae*, *Chlamydia trachomatis*, *Mycoplasma genitalium* and *Trichomonas vaginalis*. *APMIS* **2015**, *123*, 879–886. [CrossRef]
80. Kriesel, J.D.; Bhatia, A.S.; Barrus, C.; Vaughn, M.; Gardner, J.; Crisp, R.J. Multiplex PCR testing for nine different sexually transmitted infections. *Int. J. STD. AIDS* **2016**, *27*, 1275–1282. [CrossRef]
81. Choe, H.S.; Lee, D.S.; Lee, S.J.; Hong, S.H.; Park, D.C.; Lee, M.K.; Kim, T.H.; Cho, Y.H. Performance of Anyplex™ II multiplex real-time PCR for the diagnosis of seven sexually transmitted infections: Comparison with currently available methods. *Int. J. Infect. Dis.* **2013**, *17*, e1134–40. [CrossRef]
82. Berçot, B.; Amarsy, R.; Goubard, A.; Aparicio, C.; Loeung, H.U.; Segouin, C.; Gueret, H.; Jacquier, F.; Meunier, F.; Mougari, E.; et al. Assessment of coinfection of sexually transmitted pathogen microbes by use of the anyplex II STI-7 molecular kit. *J. Clin. Microbiol.* **2015**, *53*, 991–993. [CrossRef]
83. Bignell, C.; Unemo, M. European STI Guidelines Editorial Board. 2012 European guideline on the diagnosis and treatment of gonorrhoea in adults. *Int. J. STD. AIDS* **2013**, *24*, 85–92. [CrossRef]
84. Guy, R.J.; Causer, L.M.; Klausner, J.D.; Unemo, M.; Toskin, I.; Azzini, A.M.; Peeling, R.W. Performance and operational characteristics of point-of-care tests for the diagnosis of urogenital gonococcal infections. *Sex Transm. Infect.* **2017**, *93*, S16–S21. [CrossRef]
85. Abbai, N.S.; Moodley, P.; Reddy, T.; Zondi, T.G.; Rambaran, S.; Naidoo, K.; Ramjee, G. Clinical evaluation of the OneStep Gonorrhea RapiCard InstaTest for detection of *Neisseria gonorrhoeae* in symptomatic patients from KwaZulu-Natal, South Africa. *J. Clin. Microbiol.* **2015**, *53*, 1348–1350. [CrossRef]
86. Benzaken, A.S.; Galban, E.G.; Antunes, W.; Dutra, J.C.; Peeling, R.W.; Mabey, D.; Salama, A. Diagnosis of gonococcal infection in high risk women using a rapid test. *Sex Transm. Infect.* **2006**, *82* (Suppl. 5), v26–v28. [CrossRef]
87. Suzuki, K.; Matsumoto, T.; Murakami, H.; Tateda, K.; Ishii, N.; Yamaguchi, K. Evaluation of a rapid antigen detection test for *Neisseria gonorrhoeae* in urine sediment for diagnosis of gonococcal urethritis in males. *J. Infect. Chemother.* **2004**, *10*, 208–211. [CrossRef]
88. Nuñez-Forero, L.; Moyano-Ariza, L.; Gaitán-Duarte, H.; Ángel-Müller, E.; Ruiz-Parra, A.; González, P.; Rodríguez, A.; Tolosa, J.E. Diagnostic accuracy of rapid tests for sexually transmitted infections in symptomatic women. *Sex Transm. Infect.* **2016**, *92*, 24–28. [CrossRef]
89. Samarawickrama, A.; Cheserem, E.; Graver, M.; Wade, J.; Alexander, S.; Ison, C. Pilot study of use of the BioStar Optical ImmunoAssay GC point-of-care test for diagnosing gonorrhoea in men attending a genitourinary medicine clinic. *J. Med. Microbiol.* **2014**, *63*, 1111–1112. [CrossRef]
90. Peeling, R.W.; Holmes, K.K.; Mabey, D.; Ronald, A. Rapid tests for sexually transmitted infections (STIs): The way forward. *Sex Transm. Infect.* **2006**, *82*, v1–v6. [CrossRef]
91. Gaydos, C.A.; van der Pol, B.; Jett-Goheen, M.; Barnes, M.; Quinn, N.; Clark, C.; Daniel, G.E.; Dixon, P.B.; Hook, E.W., III; CT/NG Study Group. Performance of the Cepheid CT/ NG Xpert Rapid PCR Test for Detection of *Chlamydia trachomatis* and *Neisseria gonorrhoeae*. *J. Clin. Microbiol.* **2013**, *51*, 1666–1672. [CrossRef]
92. Gaydos, C.A. Review of use of a new rapid real-time PCR, the Cepheid GeneXpert®(Xpert) CT/NG assay, for *Chlamydia trachomatis* and *Neisseria gonorrhoeae*: Results for patients while in a clinical setting. *Expert. Rev. Mol. Diagn.* **2014**, *14*, 135–137. [CrossRef]
93. Garrett, N.; Mitchev, N.; Osman, F.; Naidoo, J.; Dorward, J.; Singh, R.; Ngobese, H.; Rompalo, A.; Mlisana, K.; Mindel, A. Diagnostic accuracy of the Xpert CT/NG and OSOM *Trichomonas* Rapid assays for point-of-care STI testing among young women in South Africa: A cross-sectional study. *BMJ Open* **2019**, *9*, e026888. [CrossRef]

94. Dize, L.; Silver, B.; Gaydos, C. Comparison of the Cepheid GeneXpert CT/NG assay to the Hologic Aptima Combo2 assay for the detection of *Chlamydia trachomatis* and *Neisseria gonorrhoeae* in self-collected rectal swabs. *Diagn. Microbiol. Infect. Dis.* **2018**, *90*, 83–84. [CrossRef]
95. Geiger, R.; Smith, D.M.; Little, S.J.; Mehta, S.R. Validation of the GeneXpert(R) CT/NG Assay for use with Male Pharyngeal and Rectal Swabs. *Austin. J. HIV. AIDS Res.* **2016**, *3*, 1021.
96. Murtagh, M.M. The Point-of-Care Diagnostic Landscape for Sexually Transmitted Infections (STIs). WHO, 2019. Available online: https://www.who.int/reproductivehealth/topics/rtis/Diagnostic-Landscape-for-STIs-2019.pdf (accessed on 30 January 2020).
97. Horst, A.L.; Rosenbohm, J.M.; Kolluri, N.; Hardick, J.; Gaydos, C.A.; Cabodi, M.; Klapperich, C.M.; Linnes, J.C. A paperfluidic platform to detect *Neisseria gonorrhoeae* in clinical samples. *Biomed. Microdevices* **2018**, *20*, 35. [CrossRef]
98. Harding-Esch, E.M.; Fuller, S.S.; Chow, S.L.; Nori, A.V.; Harrison, M.A.; Parker, M.; Piepenburg, O.; Forrest, M.S.; Brooks, D.G.; Patel, R.; et al. Diagnostic accuracy of a prototype rapid chlamydia and gonorrhoea recombinase polymerase amplification assay: A multicentre cross-sectional preclinical evaluation. *Clin. Microbiol. Infect.* **2019**, *25*, 380.e1–380.e7. [CrossRef]
99. Chin, C.D.; Laksanasopin, T.; Cheung, Y.K.; Steinmiller, D.; Linder, V.; Parsa, H.; Wang, J.; Moore, H.; Rouse, R.; Umviligihozo, G.; et al. Microfluidics-based diagnostics of infectious diseases in the developing world. *Nat. Med.* **2011**, *17*, 1015–1019. [CrossRef]
100. Tsaloglou, M.N.; Nemiroski, A.; Camci-Unal, G.; Christodouleas, D.C.; Murray, L.P.; Connelly, J.T.; Whitesides, G.M. Handheld isothermal amplification and electrochemical detection of DNA in resource-limited settings. *Anal. Biochem.* **2018**, *543*, 116–121. [CrossRef]
101. Unemo, M.; Shafer, W.M. Antimicrobial resistance in *Neisseria gonorrhoeae* in the 21st century: Past, evolution, and future. *Clin. Microbiol. Rev.* **2014**, *27*, 587–613. [CrossRef]
102. Donà, V.; Low, N.; Golparian, D.; Unemo, M. Recent advances in the development and use of molecular tests to predict antimicrobial resistance in *Neisseria gonorrhoeae*. *Expert. Rev. Mol. Diagn.* **2017**, *17*, 845–859. [CrossRef]
103. Peterson, S.W.; Martin, I.; Demczuk, W.; Bharat, A.; Hoang, L.; Wylie, J.; Allen, V.; Lefebvre, B.; Tyrrell, G.; Horsman, G.; et al. Molecular assay for detection of ciprofloxacin resistance in *Neisseria gonorrhoeae* isolates from cultures and clinical nucleic acid amplification test specimens. *J. Clin. Microbiol.* **2015**, *53*, 3606–3608. [CrossRef]
104. Pond, M.J.; Hall, C.L.; Miari, V.F.; Cole, M.; Laing, K.G.; Jagatia, H.; Harding-Esch, E.; Monahan, I.M.; Planche, T.; Hinds, J.; et al. Accurate detection of *Neisseria gonorrhoeae* ciprofloxacin susceptibility directly from genital and extragenital clinical samples: Towards genotype-guided antimicrobial therapy. *J. Antimicrob. Chemother.* **2016**, *71*, 897–902. [CrossRef]
105. Siedner, M.J.; Pandori, M.; Castro, L.; Barry, P.; Whittington, W.L.; Liska, S.; Klausner, J.D. Real-time PCR assay for detection of quinolone- resistant *Neisseria gonorrhoeae* in urine samples. *J. Clin. Microbiol.* **2007**, *45*, 1250–1254. [CrossRef]
106. Trembizki, E.; Buckley, C.; Donovan, B.; Chen, M.; Guy, R.; Kaldor, J.; Lahra, M.M.; Regan, D.G.; Smith, H.; Ward, J.; et al. Direct real-time PCR-based detection of *Neisseria gonorrhoeae* 23S rRNA mutations associated with azithromycin resistance. *J. Antimicrob. Chemother.* **2015**, *70*, 3244–3249. [CrossRef]
107. Ochiai, S.; Ishiko, H.; Yasuda, M.; Deguchi, T. Rapid detection of the mosaic structure of the *Neisseria gonorrhoeae* penA gene, which is associated with decreased susceptibilities to oral cephalosporins. *J. Clin. Microbiol.* **2008**, *46*, 1804–1810. [CrossRef]
108. Goire, N.; Freeman, K.; Lambert, S.B.; Nimmo, G.R.; Limnios, A.E.; Lahra, M.M.; Nissen, M.D.; Sloots, T.P.; Whiley, D.M. The influence of target population on nonculture-based detection of markers of *Neisseria gonorrhoeae* antimicrobial resistance. *Sex Health* **2012**, *9*, 422–429. [CrossRef]
109. Peterson, S.W.; Martin, I.; Demczuk, W.; Bharat, A.; Hoang, L.; Wylie, J.; Lefebvre, B.; Tyrrell, G.; Horsman, G.; Haldane, D.; et al. Molecular assay for detection of genetic markers associated with decreased susceptibility to cephalosporins in *Neisseria gonorrhoeae*. *J. Clin. Microbiol.* **2015**, *53*, 2042–2048. [CrossRef]
110. Trembizki, E.; Wand, H.; Donovan, B.; Chen, M.; Fairley, C.K.; Freeman, K.; Guy, R.; Kaldor, J.M.; Lahra, M.M.; Lawrence, A.; et al. The molecular epidemiology and antimicrobial resistance of *Neisseria gonorrhoeae* in Australia: A nationwide cross-sectional study, 2012. *Clin. Infect. Dis.* **2016**, *63*, 1591–1598. [CrossRef]

111. Donà, V.; Kasraian, S.; Lupo, A.; Guilarte, Y.N.; Hauser, C.; Furrer, H.; Unemo, M.; Low, N.; Endimiani, A. Multiplex real-time PCR assay with high-resolution melting analysis for characterization of antimicrobial resistance in *Neisseria gonorrhoeae*. *J. Clin. Microbiol.* **2016**, *54*, 2074–2081. [CrossRef]
112. Balashov, S.; Mordechai, E.; Adelson, M.E.; Gygax, S.E. Multiplex bead suspension array for screening *Neisseria gonorrhoeae* antibiotic resistance genetic determinants in noncultured clinical samples. *J. Mol. Diagn.* **2013**, *15*, 116–129. [CrossRef]
113. Donà, V.; Smid, J.H.; Kasraian, S.; Egli-Gany, D.; Dost, F.; Imeri, F.; Unemo, M.; Low, N.; Endimiani, A. Mismatch Amplification Mutation Assay-Based Real-Time PCR for Rapid Detection of *Neisseria gonorrhoeae* and Antimicrobial Resistance Determinants in Clinical Specimens. *J. Clin. Microbiol.* **2018**, *56*, e00365–18. [CrossRef]
114. Low, N.; Unemo, M. Molecular tests for the detection of antimicrobial resistant *Neisseria gonorrhoeae*: When, where, and how to use? *Curr. Opin. Infect. Dis.* **2016**, *29*, 45–51. [CrossRef]
115. Goire, N.; Lahra, M.M.; Chen, M.; Donovan, B.; Fairley, C.K.; Guy, R.; Kaldor, J.; Regan, D.; Ward, J.; Nissen, M.D.; et al. Molecular approaches to enhance surveillance of gonococcal antimicrobial resistance. *Nat. Rev. Microbiol.* **2014**, *12*, 223–229. [CrossRef]
116. Allan-Blitz, L.T.; Klausner, J.D. Codon 91 Gyrase A testing is necessary and sufficient to predict ciprofloxacin susceptibility in *Neisseria gonorrhoeae*. *J. Infect. Dis.* **2017**, *215*, 491. [CrossRef]
117. Goire, N.; Kundu, R.; Trembizki, E.; Buckley, C.; Hogan, T.R.; Lewis, D.A.; Branley, J.M.; Whiley, D.M.; Lahra, M.M. Mixed gonococcal infections in a high-risk population, Sydney, Australia 2015: Implications for antimicrobial resistance surveillance? *J. Antimicrob. Chemother.* **2017**, *72*, 407–409. [CrossRef]
118. Zhao, L.; Zhao, S. TaqMan real-time quantitative PCR assay for detection of fluoroquinolone-resistant *Neisseria gonorrhoeae*. *Curr. Microbiol.* **2012**, *65*, 692–695. [CrossRef]
119. Golparian, D.; Donà, V.; Sánchez-Busó, L.; Foerster, S.; Harris, S.; Endimiani, A.; Low, N.; Unemo, M. Antimicrobial resistance prediction and phylogenetic analysis of *Neisseria gonorrhoeae* isolates using the Oxford Nanopore MinION sequencer. *Sci. Rep.* **2018**, *8*, 17596. [CrossRef]
120. Eyre, D.W.; Golparian, D.; Unemo, M. Prediction of Minimum Inhibitory Concentrations of Antimicrobials for *Neisseria gonorrhoeae* Using Whole-Genome Sequencing. *Methods Mol. Biol.* **2019**, *1997*, 59–76. [CrossRef]

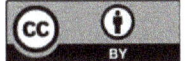

© 2020 by the authors. Licensee MDPI, Basel, Switzerland. This article is an open access article distributed under the terms and conditions of the Creative Commons Attribution (CC BY) license (http://creativecommons.org/licenses/by/4.0/).

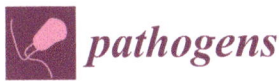

Review

Atypical, Yet Not Infrequent, Infections with *Neisseria* Species

Maria Victoria Humbert *[ID] and Myron Christodoulides

Molecular Microbiology, School of Clinical and Experimental Sciences, University of Southampton, Faculty of Medicine, Southampton General Hospital, Southampton SO16 6YD, UK; mc4@soton.ac.uk
* Correspondence: m.v.humbert@soton.ac.uk

Received: 11 November 2019; Accepted: 18 December 2019; Published: 20 December 2019

Abstract: *Neisseria* species are extremely well-adapted to their mammalian hosts and they display unique phenotypes that account for their ability to thrive within niche-specific conditions. The closely related species *N. gonorrhoeae* and *N. meningitidis* are the only two species of the genus recognized as strict human pathogens, causing the sexually transmitted disease gonorrhea and meningitis and sepsis, respectively. Gonococci colonize the mucosal epithelium of the male urethra and female endo/ectocervix, whereas meningococci colonize the mucosal epithelium of the human nasopharynx. The pathophysiological host responses to gonococcal and meningococcal infection are distinct. However, medical evidence dating back to the early 1900s demonstrates that these two species can cross-colonize anatomical niches, with patients often presenting with clinically-indistinguishable infections. The remaining *Neisseria* species are not commonly associated with disease and are considered as commensals within the normal microbiota of the human and animal nasopharynx. Nonetheless, clinical case reports suggest that they can behave as opportunistic pathogens. In this review, we describe the diversity of the genus *Neisseria* in the clinical context and raise the attention of microbiologists and clinicians for more cautious approaches in the diagnosis and treatment of the many pathologies these species may cause.

Keywords: *Neisseria* species; *Neisseria meningitidis*; *Neisseria gonorrhoeae*; commensal; pathogenesis; host adaptation

1. Introduction

The genus *Neisseria* is comprised of Gram-negative, *Betaproteobacteria* species belonging to the family *Neisseriaceae*, order *Neisseriales*. To date, about 30 *Neisseria* species have been reported (https://pubmlst.org/bigsdb?db=pubmlst_neisseria_isolates). These species are thought to be restricted to humans generally, although some have been isolated from other mammals or environmental sources [1]. Most of these organisms colonize mucosal surfaces, usually without causing overt pathology, and are therefore regarded as components of the host normal microbiota [2]. However, two species have evolved to cause disease in humans and, as such, are the only two human-restricted pathogens of the genus: *Neisseria gonorrhoeae* and *N. meningitidis* [3]. These two microorganisms are closely related and yet highly adapted to their respective host niches, causing entirely different clinical pathologies [4].

N. gonorrhoeae (the gonococcus) is an obligate pathogen that primarily colonizes the mucosal epithelium of the male urethra and female endo/ectocervix, causing the sexually transmitted disease gonorrhea. The gonococcus was discovered by Albert L. Neisser, who in 1879 described the presence of characteristic micrococci in gonorrheal pus from male and female patients [5]. Clinical symptoms for gonococcal genital infection develop as a consequence of neutrophil influx at the sites of mucosal colonization [6]. In men, infection of the urethra causes urethritis and painful discharge, and in women, localized infection of the ectocervix and endocervix leads to a mucopurulent cervicitis. However, clinical symptoms in women are more likely to go unnoticed because neutrophil infiltration does not affect the same niche as urination and pain is often absent. Although ecto/endo-cervicitis in women is commonly asymptomatic, several studies report that asymptomatic infections are indeed common in both genders [6–9]. In approximately 10–25% of untreated women, gonococci can ascend into the upper reproductive tract (through the endometrium, uterus, Fallopian tubes to ovaries and peritoneum). The host response to this ascending infection can manifest as the clinical syndrome of Pelvic Inflammatory Disease, which can leave patients with long-term and/or permanent sequelae such as chronic pelvic pain, Fallopian tube damage, endometritis, ectopic pregnancy, and infertility [6,10]. These outcomes impact significantly on the health of women worldwide.

Gonococcal infections are mainly localized in the genitourinary tract, but atypical infections can occur at other anatomical sites, as a consequence of Disseminated Gonococcal Infection (DGI), which occurs rarely, or as primary infections due to direct interaction of the pathogen. Treatment of gonorrhea has relied on antibiotics since the first introduction of penicillin in the 1940s, but this and each subsequent antibiotic class introduced has failed to treat gonococcal infections for long, due to the remarkable ability of gonococci to rapidly develop resistance. Worryingly, gonococci resistant to last-resort antibiotics are circulating now and compromising treatment. Thus, the pathogen is on the World Health Organization (WHO) 'high priority' list for research into discovering and developing new antimicrobials (https://www.who.int/medicines/publications/WHO-PPL-Short_Summary_25Feb-ET_NM_WHO.pdf). Furthermore, there are no vaccines for gonorrhea. Vaccine development remains a considerable challenge and it is still in "advanced early stage R&D" (https://vaccinesforamr.org/).

The presence of *N. gonorrhoeae* is indicative of infection, as gonococci are not part of the normal microbiota of the urogenital mucosa. Furthermore, colonization without inflammation is not considered commensalism, but an asymptomatic infection instead [3]. However, how far away is the gonococcus from being considered a commensal organism? Commensalism (literally 'to eat at the same table') is one form of symbiosis, a biological relationship between two organisms of different species, where one organism benefits while the other is generally unaffected. An organism existing in a commensal state should not elicit a vigorous and sustained host response, since host damage would not provide any selective advantage. *N. gonorrhoeae* has co-evolved with its human host for a long time, which might have resulted in a reduced/modulated pathogenic potential that benefits gonococcal replication and survival and avoids clearance [3,6]. The gonococcus has evolved several mechanisms to enable it to evade recognition and attack from human innate and adaptive immune systems [6,10]. Gonococci can survive and persist in the host using immunosuppressive mechanisms such as binding and inactivating components of the complement cascade [11,12], sialylating its lipo-oligosaccharide (LOS) to hide from the complement system [3,13] and also adapting to changing oxygen and nutrient concentrations [6,14,15]. Furthermore, although asymptomatic infection increases the possibility of complications, it promotes efficient sexual transmission from unaware individuals [6].

N. meningitidis (the meningococus) is a commensal of the human nasopharyngeal microbiota that has the potential to become invasive and cause cerebrospinal meningitis and septicemia, with significant mortality and morbidity worldwide [16]. Therefore, it might be more appropriate to describe *N. meningitidis* as an opportunistic pathogen, rather than as a commensal. The *Diplococcus intracellularis meningitidis* was discovered by Anton Weichselbaum in 1887 in the cerebrospinal fluid of patients with 'epidemic cerebrospinal meningitis' [17,18] and it was later classified as a member of the genus *Neisseria*. Today, the biology of meningococcal asymptomatic carriage and the genetic basis for the observed virulence of some disease isolates is still a matter of investigation [19]. The clinical symptoms induced by meningococcal infection reflect unrestrained compartmentalized intravascular and intracranial bacterial growth and host inflammation. Systemic (Invasive) Meningococcal Disease (SMD) can be classified into four distinctive disorders: i) Shock without meningitis (fulminant septicemia), ii) shock and meningitis, iii) meningitis without shock, and iv) meningococcemia without shock or meningitis (mild SMD, where patients usually present with fever and may also have a petechial rash) [20].

The most common presentation of SMD is meningitis, whilst fulminant meningococcal septicemia has the highest mortality rate [21]. However, other atypical, but frequent, infections can be manifested, which may sometimes be independent of preceding septicemia and mistaken also for other more common infections associated with different bacterial pathogens [21–24].

Worldwide, there are ~87 million cases of gonorrhea reported annually with the highest burden in low-to-middle income countries [25]. This is probably an underestimate due to unreported asymptomatic infections. By contrast, the cases of SMD have fallen dramatically. Based on data from the recent Global Meningococcal Initiative meeting on preventing meningococcal disease worldwide [26], a crude calculation of recent global case numbers can be made from the case incidence per 100,000 population for countries reporting infections. Globally, the number of cases can be estimated at ~14,000, and this low number is due to the dramatic reduction in cases of serogroup A disease in the 'meningitis belt' countries of sub-Saharan Africa. The burden of SMD has always been in the 'meningitis belt' and prior to introduction of MenAfriVac, the incidence of SMD cases was ~100/100,000, which equated to ~300,000–600,000 cases annually (depending on population estimates). By contrast to the typical infections of gonorrhea and SMD, the case numbers for atypical infections with *Neisseria* spp. are not known and difficult to estimate in global numbers. Moreover, any estimates of the true burden of these atypical infections are probably underestimates, due to misdiagnoses. Nevertheless, the increased number of published case reports suggests that atypical infections are rising, e.g., in cases of urogenital meningococcal infections, which can be attributed to changing sexual behaviors, notably the increased practice of oral sex has allowed *N. meningitidis* to colonize a new niche (see Section 3.1).

In general, *Neisseria* species are believed to be extremely well adapted to their primary host colonization niches and lacking the plasticity to adapt to alternative niches. It is a reasonable assumption that particular genetic features account for their unique phenotypes, their virulence potential (i.e., the development of accidental versus obligate pathogenicity) and their ability to adapt to their corresponding niche-specific conditions. The molecular bases for these qualities have yet to be wholly elucidated [4,27]. However, isolation of both gonococci and meningococci from sites other than their corresponding natural niches has been reported time and again [28–32]. In addition, infections with commensal *Neisseria* species behaving as opportunistic pathogens have been described, with the oldest reports dating to the beginning of the C20th (extensively reviewed in [33]). In this current review, we provide readers with a broad scenario of 'atypical' *Neisseria* infections, with the aim to explore the biological complexity of the genus and raise awareness of these apparently not uncommon events, which may lead to misdiagnosis and consequent inappropriate/ineffective medical treatment. A glossary for the medical terms used throughout this review is provided in Table S1.

2. Atypical Infections with *N. gonorrhoeae*

2.1. Disseminated Gonococcal Infections (DGIs)

Along with complications from untreated, ascending, female genital tract infections, gonococci can, on rare occasions, enter the bloodstream and cause DGI. Disseminated infection is one of the major threats of gonococcal infection, since the outcome is potentially fatal [34]. Sequelae generally associated with DGI are infectious arthritis, rash, endocarditis or meningitis, resulting mainly from blood dissemination of *N. gonorrhoeae* from primary sexually acquired mucosal infection [35,36]. DGI should also be suspected on appearance of tenosynovitis, polyarthralgia and skin lesions, although these clinical presentations are more commonly associated with gonococcal bacteremia [37].

Neurological manifestations of gonorrhea were observed possibly as early as 1805 by Home [38,39]; however, the first definite case of meningitis attributable to *N. gonorrhoeae* was reported in 1922 [40]. Furthermore, *N. gonorrhoeae* was first implicated as a potential cause of endocarditis by Ricord in 1834 [41,42], but it was not until 1895 that Thayer and Blumer were able to recover this organism from the blood and from lesions on the affected valves of a patient with apparent endocarditis [42,43]. A second case of septicemia with subsequent ulcerative endocarditis due to gonococcal infection was reported in 1899 [44] (Table 1). Despite DGI being a rare complication, its incidence is currently increasing relative to the steady increase in the incidence of gonorrhea worldwide [45].

Table 1. Examples of reported clinical cases of unusual infections with *Neisseria* species.

Neisseria species	Anatomical Site of Infection	Disease	Case Report
		Pathogenic *Neisseria* species	
N. gonorrhoeae [1]	Blood	DGI/septicemia	[34,43,44,46–49]
	Joints	DGI/arthritis	[35,37]
	Heart	DGI/endocarditis	[42–45,50]
	Skin (extragenital)	DGI/cutaneous infection	[51–53]
	Brain	DGI/meningitis	[38–40,54]
	Pharynx	DGI/pharyngitis	[55]
		Oro- and nasopharyngeal infections	[32,56–62]
		Tonsillitis	[63]
	Mouth/lips	Stomatitis	
	Parotid glands	Parotitis	[64]
	Tendon	DGI/tenosynovitis	[61]
	Eye	Keratoconjunctivitis	[31,65]
		Conjunctivitis/*ophthalmia neonatorum*	[49,62,66–72]
	Scalp	Scalp abscess	[73]
	Breast	Mastitis/breast abscess	[74–77]
N. meningitidis [2]	Genitourinary tract	Vaginitis	[29,78–81]
		Urethritis	[30,82–94]
		Cervicitis	[78,79,83,85,86,89,90,93,95–98]
		Anal canal infection/proctitis	[83,86,88–90]
		Intrauterine infection	[99]
	Eye	Conjunctivitis	[81,97,100–111]
		Endophthalmitis	[112–120]
		Panophthalmitis	[121]
		Commensal *Neisseria* species [3]	
N. bacilliformis	Heart	Endocarditis	[122,123]
	Oral cavity/fistula	Submandibular wound	[124]
	Sputum	Possible bronchitis	[124]
	Sputa	Possible bronchitis	[124]
	Lung	Lung abscess	[124]
	Blood	(Insufficient clinical data)	[124]
N. canis	Lung	Bronchiectasis	[125]
	Skin	Purulent wound/cellulitis	[126]
N. cinerea	Blood	Septicemia	[127,128]
	Brain	Meningitis	[128]
	Genitourinary tract	Genital infections	[129]
		Urinary infection	[130]
	Peritoneum	Peritonitis	[131]
	Eye	Conjunctivitis/*ophthalmia neonatorum*	[132,133]
N. dumasiana	Sputum	(Insufficient clinical data)	[134]

Table 1. Cont.

Neisseria species	Anatomical Site of Infection	Disease	Case Report
Commensal Neisseria species [3]			
N. elongata	Heart	Endocarditis	[135,136]
	Blood	Septicemia	[137]
	Bone	Osteomyelitis	[138]
N. flava	Heart	Rheumatic heart disease/ventricular septaldefect/endocarditis	[139]
		Endocarditis	[140]
	Blood	Sepsis/conjunctival petechia	[139]
N. flavescens	Heart	Endocarditis	[141,142]
	Brain	Meningitis	[143,144]
	Blood	Septicemia	[145,146]
	Lung	Pneumonia/empyema	[147]
	Genitourinary tract	Genital infections	[148]
N. lactamica	Brain	Meningitis	[149,150]
	Blood	Septicemia	[145,151]
	Pharynx	Pharyngitis	[152]
	Lung	Cavitary lesion	[153]
		Pneumonia	[154]
	Genitourinary tract	Genital infections	[129,155,156]
N. mucosa	Heart	Endocarditis	[157–159]
	Brain	Meningitis	[160,161]
	Blood	Septicemia	[145,162]
	Lung	Empyema	[163]
	Genitourinary tract	Genital infections	[129]
		Urinary infection	[164]
	Viscera	Botryomycosis	[165]
	Joints	Arthritis	[166,167]
N. oralis	Bladder	Cystitis	[168]
	Gingiva	Healthy gingival plaque/subgingival oral biofilm	[169]
	Blood	(Insufficient clinical data)	[169]
	Urinary tract	(Insufficient clinical data)	[169]
	Paracentesis fluid	(Insufficient clinical data)	[169]
N. perflava	Heart	Endocarditis	[170,171]
N. shayeganii	Sputum	(Insufficient clinical data)	[172]
	Skin	Arm wound	[172]
N. sicca	Heart	Endocarditis	[173–176]
	Brain	Meningitis	[177,178]
	Blood	Septicemia	[145]
	Lung	Pneumonia	[179]
	Genitourinary tract	Genital infections	[148,180,181]
		Urinary infection	[182]

Table 1. Cont.

Neisseria species	Anatomical Site of Infection	Disease	Case Report
N. subflava	Heart	Endocarditis	[183,184]
	Brain	Meningitis	[185–187]
	Blood	Septicemia	[145,186]
	Genitourinary tract	Genital infections	[148,180,188]
		Urinary infection	[189]
N. wadsworthii	Skin	Hand wound	[172]
	Peritoneal fluid	(Insufficient clinical data)	[172]
N. weaveri	Blood	Septicemia	[190]
	Sputum	Bronchiectasis	[191]
	Peritoneum	Peritonitis	[192]
	Skin	Wound	[193,194]
N. zoodegmatis	Skin	Ulceration	[195]

Table 1 Legend. Only exemplar clinical case reports of unusual infections with pathogenic and commensal *Neisseria* species are listed in the Table 1; characteristic (typical) infections with gonococcus (gonorrhea) and meningococcus (meningitis and septicemia) are not included. [1] Many of the unusual gonococcal infections are associated with preceding disseminated gonococcal infection (DGI) (consequential of initial gonorrhea) or serve as a portal of entry for gonococcal septicemia and/or other manifestations of DGI. [2] Some clinical cases of unusual meningococcal infections are either associated with preceding meningococcemia or further develop sepsis (systemic (invasive) meningococcal disease (SMD)) as a consequence of the corresponding primary infection. [3] Commensal *Neisseria* species are not associated with disease, although they may behave as opportunistic pathogens. In many of these cases, an overlap of clinical features for different conditions is generally observed (e.g., invasion of the bloodstream by *Neisseria* may also occur in cases of endocarditis and meningitis). The current, accepted nomenclature for the *Neisseria* species is provided in the Table 1, so the corresponding classifications for generic and specific names allocated in the oldest reports may vary (e.g., '*Micrococcus pharyngis siccus*' in reference [174] refers to *Neisseria sicca*, as stated in the Table 1). Gram-negative diplococci *Moraxella* (*Branhamella*) *catarrhalis* (formely known as *N. catarrhalis*) is a common, essentially harmless inhabitant of the pharynx, but can also behave as an opportunistic pathogen, causing infections mainly in both the upper and lower respiratory tract. Due to its high phenotypic resemblance to the Neisseriae, it was frequently confused with another pharyngeal resident, *Neisseria cinerea* [196]. With this proviso in mind, old case reports of infection with '*N. catarrhalis*' are discussed in the text but are not included in this Table 1 due to its re-classification [197].

In common with all other *Neisseria* species, gonococci do not have an enhanced ability to leave their normal colonization niches, probably due to their reduced capacity to survive systemically [3]. However, *N. gonorrhoeae* strains associated with DGI are more serum resistant than strains isolated from localized infections [46]. Although *N. gonorrhoeae* lacks a capsule polysaccharide (CPS) to protect itself against serum complement-mediated lysis and opsonophagocytosis, the organism has evolved mechanisms to evade recognition and attack from the human complement system [3,11–13]. Certain gonococcal isolates are more disposed than others to become systemic, and it is presumed that both bacterial and host factors contribute to DGI [47,48]. Indeed, a variable genetic island present in *N. gonorrhoeae* and absent in *N. meningitidis* and in all commensal *Neisseria* species, was related to an ability of DGI-associated gonococcal isolates to become systemic [198]. Particular types of this horizontally acquired collection of chromosomally localized genes, i.e., the ones carried preferentially by DGI isolates, confer *N. gonorrhoeae* with a serum resistance locus and encodes also for a peptidoglycan hydrolase that is similar to bacteriophage transglycosylases. Expression of this peptidoglycan hydrolase may correlate with increased peptidoglycan-cytotoxin production [199], thus contributing to enhanced pathogenicity and increased ability of gonococci to survive systemically. Furthermore, all of the different types of this genetic island encode homologues of F factor conjugation proteins, suggesting an involvement in a conjugation-like secretion system, providing DNA for natural transformation [198].

2.2. Gonococcal Oral and Nasopharyngeal Infections

Gonococcal nasopharyngeal infection could potentially result as a consequence of DGI [55], although it is more generally correlated to preceding orogenital contact [56]. Conversely, disseminated gonorrhea from a primary pharyngeal infection also has been described [57]. The presence of *N. gonorrhoeae* in the human pharynx is reported frequently [28,32,56,58,59,63], probably more so than meningococcal infections of the cervix or the urethra (see below, Section 3.1). Frazer and Menton reported in 1931 a rare case of gonococcal stomatitis and stated that about 40 other cases had been recorded previously since Neisser discovered the gonococcus in 1879, although with no complete proof that the gonococcus was the causative organism [200]. Copping in 1954 [201] and Schmidt et al. in 1961 [202] subsequently reported clinical cases of gonococcal stomatitis, and several other cases with similar clinical presentations have been recorded ever since [203,204]. In 1953, Diefenbach described an infection of the parotid gland with *N. gonorrhoeae* following fellatio of a man with confirmed urethral gonorrhea [64]. Fiumara et al. in 1967 described the first report of gonococcal pharyngitis [60] and two years later, in 1969, Cowan reported a case of a female patient with gonococcal cervicitis and urethritis who developed gonococcal ulceration of the tongue [52]. Today, cases of gonococcal nasopharyngeal infections are reported commonly [205]. The presence of gonococci in the pharynx correlates poorly with symptoms of sore throat [56,59], and cases of symptomatic pharyngitis may be caused by other sexually transmitted agents, particularly in those cases of preceding orogenital contact [28]. However, rare cases of symptomatic gonococcal pharyngitis have been described [61] (Table 1). Interestingly, in the UK in 2016, the first global failure of treating pharyngeal gonorrhea was reported, caused by an eXtensively Drug Resistant (XDR) gonococcus with resistance to both ceftriaxone and azithromycin [206]. Furthermore, in the UK in 2018, a case was reported of a male diagnosed with urethral and pharyngeal gonorrhea; antibiotics cured the urethral infection, but pharyngeal infection was resistant to ceftriaxone, doxycycline, and spectinomycin and finally required intravenous ertapenem for eradication [207]. The increase in pharyngeal gonorrhea is a global concern, enabling both the spread of XDR gonococci and potentially leading to untreatable infections, as drug penetration of the pharynx is poor [205].

2.3. Gonococcal Ophthalmia

N. gonorrhoeae can colonize the human ocular mucosa as an alternative site of infection. When it occurs in neonates, known as gonococcal *ophthalmia neonatorum*, transmission of *N. gonorrhoeae* and subsequent development of eye infection in the newborn often occurs during delivery and as a direct consequence of exposure to infectious vaginal secretions [66,67]. Vertical transmission of *N. gonorrhoeae* is still possible even with delivery via Caesarean section [68–70], which may also cause, although very rarely, some other complications in the neonate apart from ocular infections, such as gonococcal infection of the fetal scalp [73]. Moreover, the above symptoms worsen in cases where gonococcal scalp abscess and necrosis become a focus for disseminated infection [62] (Table 1).

Gonococcal infection of newborn eyes, although frequently mild, can be rapidly destructive and lead to corneal scarring and blindness. In severe cases, corneal ulceration ensues, with probable perforation of the globe and consequential panophthalmitis [62]. Although most cases of gonococcal *ophthalmia neonatorum* are self-limiting and generally benign with appropriate treatment, the infected conjunctivae occasionally serve as a portal of entry for gonococci to induce septicemia, meningitis, arthritis, and/or other manifestations of DGI [49,54] (Table 1).

While typically thought of as a disease in neonates, gonococcal conjunctivitis is an issue also for other age groups. The infection is still reported infrequently in adults and transmission of *N. gonorrhoeae* generally occurs via direct sexual contact with infective secretions [71,72] (Table 1). Indirect transmission, e.g., manually or via fomites, is thought to be less likely, since the microorganism does not survive for long outside its human host. Unlike more common forms of bacterial conjunctivitis in adults, gonococcal infection can cause corneal perforation requiring surgical repair which, if left untreated, could lead to permanent blindness within hours [65,208]. Therefore, rapid arrest of the disease in adults is also essential.

2.4. Gonococcal Mastitis

Mastitis is infectious or non-infectious inflammation of the breast, and mastitis caused by *N. gonorrhoeae* infection is extremely rare. Gonococcal mastitis was first reported in the literature in 1993 [74] and only three other similar clinical cases have been described since [75–77]. All of the patients in these cases had healed nipple piercings prior to oral-nipple contact, and no other organisms were isolated. *N. gonorrhoeae* cutaneous abscesses in non-genital sites, such as the abdomen, hand, and fetal scalp, have been associated initially with DGI, secondary to disseminated disease [53]. However, other than by hematogenous metastasis from the site of a primary infection, gonococcal abscesses can also occur as a result of direct inoculation or local spread and are often preceded by skin barrier breakdown. This is the case for all four reports of gonococcal mastitis, where the presence of a piercing probably disrupted the skin barrier, predisposing to abscess formation upon exposure to the organism [74–77] (Table 1).

3. Atypical Infections with *N. meningitidis*

3.1. Meningococcal Genitourinary Tract Infections

N. gonorrhoeae and *Chlamydia trachomatis* are the two most common pathogens colonizing the male and female urogenital tract mucosa [209]. However, *N. meningitidis* can be sporadically pathogenic in the genitourinary tract, as first reported by Murray in 1939 [82]. In several subsequent reports, the presence of *N. meningitidis* in the urethra was not associated with genital symptoms [78,83,84,95]. However, genital infections caused by meningococci may sometimes present similar clinical symptoms to classical gonorrhea, e.g., purulent penile discharge and urethritis, and cervicitis/vaginitis [29,30,85–87,93,94] (Table 1).

A recent analysis of urogenital and rectal infections revealed co-colonization with encapsulated, hyperinvasive meningococci and closely related MultiDrug-Resistant (MDR) gonococci [88]. The main concern with co-infection is an increased chance that meningococci acquire gonococcal antimicrobial resistance genes. Co-existence of meningococci with gonococci poses a clear risk to public health, as the emergence of menincococcal strains with expanded antimicrobial resistance could contribute to therapeutic complications in the treatment of meningococcal disease. In fact, urogenital meningococcal isolates possessing gonococcal plasmids have been described [89]. Furthermore, expansion of a US non-groupable (unencapsulated) urethritis-associated *N. meningitidis* clade (NmNG) with concurrent acquisition of *N. gonorrhoeae* alleles has been reported recently [90,91]. However, acquisition of common gonococcal antimicrobial resistance factors by this clade has not been described to date. Nonetheless, in the study from Retchless et al. [90], the authors suggested that since the clinical presentation of meningococcal urethritis mirrors that of gonococcal infections, 'the evolutionary forces that resulted in high rates of antimicrobial resistance among *N. gonorrhoeae* may lead to the same result among these *N. meningitidis*'.

The reasons why a commensal organism of the human nasopharynx may become pathogenic and the molecular mechanisms that perturb the host-bacterium equilibrium are mostly unknown. A whole-genome comparison of disease and carriage meningococcal strains provided insights into the virulence evolution of *N. meningitidis* and it suggested that this bacterium emerged as an encapsulated human commensal from a common ancestor with *N. gonorrhoeae* and *N. lactamica*, subsequently acquiring the genes responsible for capsule synthesis via horizontal gene transfer [16]. The *cps* locus required for capsule synthesis consists of several regions, some of which might belong to the *Neisseria* core genome because they can be found in many other *Neisseria* spp. However, the regions containing the genes required for capsule synthesis, modification, and transport can be found only in the encapsulated meningococcal strains [16]. Some of these genes are highly similar in sequence and operon organization to homologous genes in the *Pasteurella multocida* genome [16]. These observations are in line with previous studies reporting horizontal gene transfer from encapsulated *Haemophilus influenzae* (a member of the *Pasteurellaceae* and a resident of the human airways) to *N. meningitidis* [210].

Thus, horizontal gene transfer between different bacterial species present in the oro-nasopharyngeal microbiota may drive evolutionary events.

Expression of capsule is the only feature that has been linked convincingly to the pathogenic potential of *N. meningitidis*: capsule mediates protection from desiccation during transmission and mediates resistance against complement-mediated lysis and opsonophagocytosis during SMD [211–216]. However, although meningococcal carriage isolates are frequently unencapsulated due to absence of the genetic island encoding for capsule synthesis [217], carriage isolates expressing capsule otherwise associated with disease have been reported [218–220]. Therefore, the conclusion that the capsule is necessary, but not sufficient, to confer virulence would seem to be fair, except for those unique cases of meningococcal urethral infections with unencapsulated isolates belonging to the US NmNG clade described above [91]. Since capsule expression contributes to virulence during SMD [211], disruption of the *cps* locus in the US NmNG urethritis-associated clade was expected to limit the risk of SMD from this clade. However, five unencapsulated isolates from SMD cases were identified, and primary urethral colonization was proposed to contribute to subsequent sepsis caused by this NmNG clade [90]. These urethritis-associated isolates have adapted particularly to the urogenital environment with two unique molecular fingerprints: A multi-gene deletion at the capsule synthesis locus that enhances mucosal adherence, and acquisition of the gonococcal denitrification pathway by gene conversion that promotes anaerobic growth [92]. These phenotypic changes, and potentially others, suggest that multiple independent evolutionary events have selected this newly emergent lineage meningococcal clade to better assimilate into the same niche first populated by gonococci, and thus become a successful urogenital pathogen [90,92], but one that maintains its competence to cause SMD [90].

In previous studies, the route by which *N. meningitidis* reached the genital tract was highly speculative. For example, in Murray's report, the isolation of meningococci from the urogenital tract of male patients was associated with meningococcal septicemia in which the testes and epididymides were involved [82]. In two female patients described by Keys et al. [95], the presence of endocervical meningococci was also associated with meningococcemia, but it was unclear whether meningococcemia preceded cervical infection, or vice versa. In the majority of other cases described in the literature, however, patients from whom meningococci were isolated from the cervix or the urethra, did not present any signs of septicemia, and it seems unlikely that the organism reached the genital tract by the hematogenous route. In the majority of these cases, transmission by orogenital sexual activity seems probable [28,29,78,84,85]. Several cases of neonatal meningococcal meningitis associated with maternal cervical-vaginal colonization have also been reported [79,80,99], with the first report in 1997 by Harriau et al. of associated oropharyngeal colonization of the male partner [96]. In this study, the phenotypic and genomic identities of meningococcal strains isolated from both the endocervix of the infected pregnant woman and her male partner was the first clear evidence for *N. meningitidis* cross-colonization between sexual partners. In addition, the possibility of self-transmission from the pharynx to the urethra via the hands also certainly exists, as suggested by a case report of a male heterosexual patient who harbored organisms of the same serotype and sensitivity patterns in both sites [28] (Table 1).

3.2. Meningococcal Ophthalmia

By contrast to gonococcal infections of the eye [6], meningococcal eye infections are more rare. Since *N. gonorrhoeae* and *N. meningitidis* cannot be differentiated with Gram's stain, because they both appear as Gram-negative diplococci [221], clinical symptoms of apparent gonococcal ocular infections should be approached with caution so as not to misdiagnose the odd cases of meningococcal *ophthalmia*, which may develop further into more severe sequelae. Meningococcal conjunctivitis is a rare condition that can have devastating ocular and systemic complications, and hence topical antibiotics alone are insufficient for treatment [100,101]. Simple conjunctivitis can progress into endophthalmitis, which is accompanied usually by severe pain, loss of vision, and redness of the conjunctiva and the underlying episclera. Meningococcal endophthalmitis presents variably with sepsis [102,112,113,121], meningitis [114,115], or isolated ocular symptoms without systemic illness [112,116–119], although subsequent development of other expressions of meningococcal disease should not be ruled out [103–105]. Thus, delayed or incorrect treatment of meningococcal ocular infections ultimately risks blindness, disability, or death [120] (Table 1).

Natural populations of *N. meningitidis* carried in the nasopharynx are not associated with invasive disease [217], and yet retain the potential to become pathogenic by entering the bloodstream, crossing the blood–cerebrospinal fluid barrier (BCSFB) and invading the meninges [222]. Invasion of the BCSFB and blood–ocular barriers by meningococci suggests common antigenic expression in meningeal and ocular microvascular endothelial beds. The possibility of meningococci reaching the ocular site by the hematogenous route is feasible but unproven [103]. Indeed, meningococcal ocular infections are most commonly associated with preceding SMD and rarely occur in isolation. Nonetheless, cases of primary meningococcal conjunctivitis (with no associated symptoms of SMD) resulting from close contact with another patient diagnosed with meningitis [101] and even through transmission from direct ocular contact with saliva from apparently healthy individuals [106,107], suggest that the routes of transmission to the eye may differ in each particular clinical case (Table 1).

Unusual cases of neonatal meningococcal conjunctivitis have also been reported. The first report of primary neonatal meningococcal conjunctivitis is from Hansman and dates back to 1972 [108]. In this study, the source of infection was not established, since cultures of cervical and urethral swabs collected from the mother failed to yield *Neisseria* (Table 1). Hansman therefore considered that the neonatal infection probably originated by contact with a different meningococcal carrier, possibly a member of the hospital staff. Subsequently, other cases of primary meningococcal conjunctivitis in newborn infants acquired by direct contact with an exogenous meningococcal source have been described [109]. More recently, an unusual case of vertical transmission of *N. meningitidis* to a neonate acquired at delivery, with subsequent development of neonatal primary meningococcal conjunctivitis, was reported by Fiorito et al. [97]. In this report, the source of transmission to the neonate was confirmed to be the mother's endocervical infection (see above, Section 3.1), and sexual cross-transmission of the same strain with her partner was also proved [97]. This case study from Fiorito et al. is the first report of an alternative transmission pathway by which *N. meningitidis* may reach and colonize the eye that is different to transmission via the hematogenous route and/or via direct contact with an exogenous source [97,110]. Meningococcal neonatal purulent conjunctivitis and consequential sepsis associated with asymptomatic carriage of *N. meningitidis* in the mother's vagina and both parents' nasopharynx has also been described [81]. In this study, it is possible that the bacteria in the newborn were acquired by vertical transmission from the mother's vagina during delivery, and the presence of bacteria in the nasopharynx of both parents suggested also horizontal transmission amongst them [81] (Table 1).

Neonatal meningococcal meningitis following meningococcal conjunctivitis, where the eye may have been the portal of entry after intrapartum contamination with the pathogen, is rare [223]. In the cases reported by Sunderland et al. in 1972 [80] and Jones et al. in 1976 [79], the ultimate outcome of disease was child death. The first report of a surviving newborn infected in the same manner was published by Ellis et al. in 1984 [111] (Table 1). Thus, quick and precise diagnosis and treatment of meningococcal conjunctivitis in neonates is crucial, as inappropriate management of a primary eye infection with *N. meningitidis* may have severe implications for the newborn's health.

4. Infections with Commensal *Neisseria* Species

Non-pathogenic *Neisseria* species comprise part of the commensal bacterial microbiota of the human and animal oropharynx, but might occasionally behave as opportunistic pathogens [1,224]. Whether this commensal population contributes to human health and/or impacts on colonization and disease caused by bacterial pathogens remains to be elucidated. Kim et al. (2019) [225] reported the first clear evidence that commensal *Neisseria* can kill *N. gonorrhoeae* through a DNA-mediated mechanism based on genetic competence and DNA methylation state, accelerating clearance of gonococci in a DNA-uptake-dependent manner. Consistent with these findings, the authors suggested that the antagonistic behavior of commensal *Neisseria* toward their pathogenic relatives may negatively affect *N. gonorrhoeae* colonization and that DNA is a potential microbicidal agent against drug-resistant gonococci [225].

There is ample evidence in the literature, however, that these 'apparently harmless' inhabitants of the oropharynx are capable of producing infection in a wide variety of anatomical sites including the heart, nervous system (meningitis), bloodstream (septicemia), respiratory tract, bone marrow, skin and possibly the genital tract. Many of these infections occur possibly secondary to a primary infection elsewhere, e.g., subsequent invasion of the bloodstream by *Neisseria* from the oropharynx may lead to endocarditis and meningitis, with an overlap of the clinical features of these conditions [1,33].

4.1. Endocarditis

To our knowledge, the first recorded case of endocarditis caused by a 'presumably' commensal *Neisseria* species was probably from Coulter in 1915 [226], although the organism, referred to as a 'Gram-negative *Micrococcus*', was inadequately characterized. Regardless, Coulter's study was considered by Johnson in his literature review in 1983 on the pathogenic potential of commensal *Neisseria* species [33]. Schultz described the first confirmed case of endocarditis as a consequence of infection with a commensal species of *Neisseria* in 1918, identified as '*Micrococcus pharyngitidis-siccae*' (*N. sicca*, as we know it today) [173]. Graef et al. described a case of endocarditis caused by this same organism in 1932, but referred to it as '*Micrococcus pharyngis siccus*' [174]. Since then, many other cases of confirmed endocarditis caused by *N. sicca* have been recorded [175,176]. Other commensal *Neisseria* species have also been associated with heart infections, e.g., *N. bacilliformis* [122,123], *N. elongata* [135,136], *N. flava* [139,140], *N. flavescens* [141,142], *N. mucosa* [157–159], *N. perflava* [170,171], and *N. subflava* [183,184], (Table 1).

4.2. Meningitis and Septicemia

In 1908, Wilson described a case of cerebrospinal meningitis caused by *Micrococcus catarrhalis* (also previously described as *N. catarrhalis*, now *Moraxella (Branhamella) catarrhalis*) [227]. Since then, *Neisseria* spp. other than *N. meningitidis* and *N. gonorrhoeae* identified as causing meningitis include *N. flavescens* [143,144], *N. lactamica* [149,150], *N. mucosa* [160,161], *N. sicca* [177,178], and *N. subflava* [185–187]. Moreover, several non-gonococcal, non-meningococcal *Neisseria* species have been isolated from blood cultures, many of which have been associated with infections including endocarditis (see above, Section 4.1), septicemia and meningitis [124,127,128,137,139,145,146,151,162,169,186,190] (Table 1).

4.3. Respiratory Tract Infections

The association of *Neisseria* spp. with respiratory tract infection pathologies is challenging as *Neisseria* organisms, with the sole exception of the gonococcus, are known to inhabit harmlessly the upper respiratory tract [2]. Nevertheless, there is increasing evidence to suggest that *N. catarrhalis* (*M. catarrhalis*), can cause infections in the upper and lower respiratory tract, with associated symptoms of otitis, laryngitis, bronchitis, bronchiectasis, pneumonia, or sinusitis [228–238]. Similarly, *N. bacilliformis* [124], *N. canis* [125], *N. flavescens* [147], *N. lactamica* [152–154], *N. mucosa* [163], *N. sicca* [179], and *N. weaveri* [191], have also been reported to cause respiratory tract infections (Table 1).

4.4. Genitourinary Tract Infections

Isolation of Gram-negative diplococci from genital tract smears is generally thought to be evidence of gonococcal infection [6]. However, as discussed in Section 3.1, meningococcal genitourinary tract infections do also occur and similarly, several commensal *Neisseria* spp. have been isolated from the genitourinary tract, although it is not clear whether these organisms cause any pathological changes or symptoms when colonizing this anatomical site. Nevertheless, absence of symptomatic disease does not necessarily imply that these other *Neisseria* spp. do not have pathogenic potential, since infection with the gonococcus is frequently asymptomatic, especially in women [239]. The earliest reports of non-gonococcal, commensal *Neisseria* spp. present in the genital tract include *N. catarrhalis* (*M. catarrhalis*) [148,180,240–242], *N. flavescens* [148], *N. lactamica* [155,156], *N. sicca* [148,180,181], and *N. subflava* [148,180,188]. More recently, further examples of male genitourinary infections with *N. cinerea*, *N. lactamica*, and *N. mucosa* have been described [129] (Table 1).

4.5. Other Infections, Epidemiology, and Factors Possibly Influencing Disease Development

Since the early 1900s, numerous clinical cases have been described in the literature of commensal *Neisseria* spp. capable of colonizing a wide variety of anatomical sites other that the nasopharynx and causing disease. Thus, only exemplar reports are cited in this current review (Table 1). These cases and other pathologies associated with infection with non-pathogenic *Neisseria* spp., such us peritonitis [131,192], purulent wound and cellulitis [126], osteomyelitis [138], skin ulceration [195], visceral botryomycosis [165], neonatal conjunctivitis [132,133], and cystitis [168] have been thoroughly reviewed by Liu et al. in 2015 [1] (Table 1).

From an epidemiological perspective, infections with commensal *Neisseria* spp. occur as singular events rather than as outbreaks, except for probably one single event of epidemic meningitis caused by *N. flavescens* reported in 1930 [143]. This epidemiology suggests minimal person-to-person transmission, and development of the disease may probably be due to endogenous spread of the organism from a primary infected site (oropharynx). In this scenario, a host prone to infection (e.g., immunocompromised) and/or enhanced virulence of the particular infective strain may determine the outcome of disease, as in cases of DGI [47,48] and SMD [243]. For instance, access of the organism to the bloodstream as a direct consequence of a preceding oral trauma, such as in cases of endocarditis, meningitis and septicemia, suggests that the infective organisms should be resistant to the bactericidal activity of normal human serum. Whether 'commensal' *Neisseria* isolated from blood are serum resistant in comparison to isolates of the same species confined to the nasopharynx, remains to be elucidated. Alternatively, host immuno-deficiency may predispose susceptible individuals to systemic infections, as observed with patients suffering from DGI and SMD [244]. Furthermore, successful colonization of the anatomical site, which requires organism attachment to host cells to establish commensalism, precedes blood invasion and intravascular survival. Once established, the organism should be capable of resisting clearance by host immune defenses, perhaps through molecular mechanisms similarly described for the gonococcus [6,10,245,246]?

5. Antimicrobial Treatment of Typical and Atypical *Neisseria* Infections

Complicated gonorrhea (DGI) and meningococcal disease are both life-threatening infections that, even after initiation of appropriate treatment, may progress rapidly and be potentially fatal. Timely diagnosis is key for effective management and both are crucial to prevent or reduce the complications of infection. Thus, increased awareness is needed for i) the possibility of atypical infections with commensal *Neisseria* spp. resembling those clinical symptoms associated with *N. gonorrhoeae* and *N. meningitidis* infections, ii) the likelihood of atypical infections with these pathogens in alternative anatomical sites, and iii) knowledge on how to treat them effectively. Typical, uncomplicated gonorrhea is usually treated empirically with a short course of antibiotics, without testing for antimicrobial susceptibility. The Centers for Disease Control and Prevention (CDC) recommends a single dose of 250 mg of intramuscular ceftriaxone and 1 g of oral azithromycin (https://www.cdc.gov/std/tg2015/gonorrhea.htm). In the UK, given the rise in resistance to azithromycin, the 2019 guidelines from the British Association for Sexual Health and HIV (BASHH), recommends ceftriaxone 1 g intramuscularly as a single dose (https://www.bashhguidelines.org/current-guidelines/urethritis-and-cervicitis/gonorrhoea-2019/). For DGI, the CDC recommends a variety of antibiotics including ceftriaxone, azithromycin and cefotaxime, depending on the clinical presentation, e.g., arthritis and meningitis. Cefotaxime, ceftriaxone and benzylpenicillin are preferred as initial therapy in patients with a clinical diagnosis of SMD, although alternative antibiotic therapies to treat typical meningococcal disease are also available [247]. In general, similar antimicrobial treatments for atypical infections with *N. gonorrhoeae* and *N. meningitidis* have also proved successful (Table S2). However, antimicrobial prescription for atypical infections with commensal *Neisseria* spp. varies widely depending on the species and on the anatomical site of infection (Table S2). Therefore, precise diagnosis is essential.

6. Discussion

Neisseria spp. are highly adapted to the environmental conditions of the unique niches that they colonize. However, the genus *Neisseria* is far more diverse and complex than acknowledged previously. For example, 'commensal' *Neisseria* spp. have generally been regarded as harmless organisms of little clinical importance, but it is clear that they can occasionally disseminate from their commensal niche and occupy, survive and proliferate in other anatomical niches and cause serious infections (Figure 1) [1,33]. Conversely, the closely related pathogens of the genus, *N. gonorrhoeae* and *N. meningitidis*, have adapted evolutionarily to their specific niche and cause diseases with distinctive profiles. However, their differences can sometimes be compensated by their biological similarities, which may probably explain those cases in which these two organisms behave in clinically-indistinguishable fashion (Figure 1) [98,248].

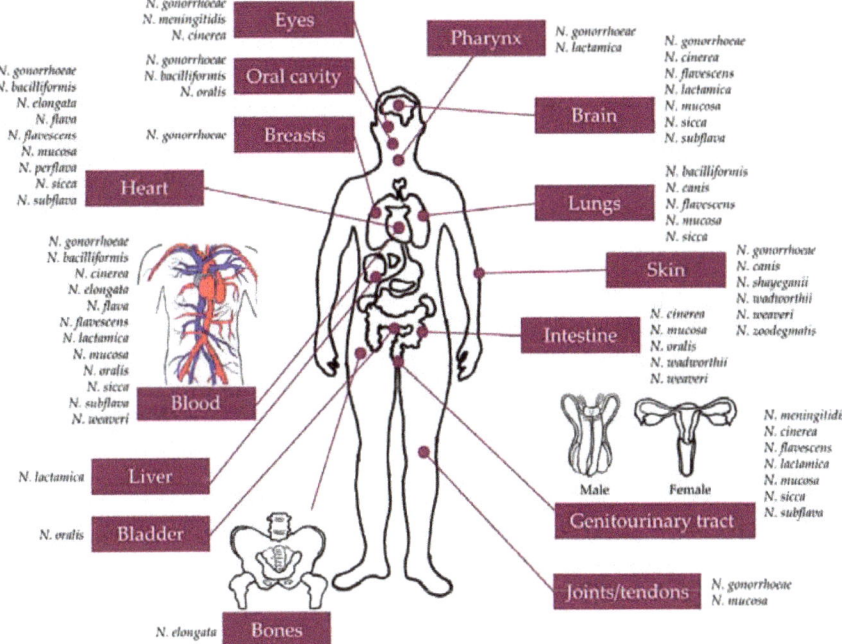

Figure 1. Legend. Only exemplar atypical anatomical sites infected by pathogenic and commensal *Neisseria* species are depicted. Corresponding references for these and other clinical case reports of unusual infections with *Neisseria* species are listed in Table 1. Characteristic (typical) infections with gonococcus (gonorrhea) and meningococcus (meningitis and septicemia) are not included. Many of the unusual gonococcal infections are either associated with preceding DGI or considered the cause of subsequent gonococcal septicemia and/or other manifestations of DGI. Some clinical cases of unusual meningococcal infections are either associated with preceding meningococcaemia or further develop sepsis (SMD) as a consequence of the corresponding primary infection (refer to the main text for more details).

Successful colonization of the mammalian host by *Neisseria* spp. requires an initial adhesive interaction between the bacterium and the host mucosal epithelial cell. *Neisseria* adhesion to the exposed epithelia depends on a repertoire of diverse molecules within the bacterial outer membrane (OM) and extending from the bacterial surface and their interplay with specific host cell receptors [249–252]. Models of *Neisseria* spp. colonization suggest that after initial adhesion, maintenance of association involves bacterial aggregation, microcolony, and biofilm formation and the activation of mechanisms to avoid host immunity [253,254]. Despite the fact that *Neisseria* spp. colonize specific, distinctive niches, ample evidence of these species adhering to and colonizing other anatomical sites, some of which are colonized by more than one species, suggests that pathogenic and commensal *Neisseria* might share conserved surface molecules important for bacterial-host cell interactions. In fact, for classical *Neisseria* infections, a great deal is known about the biology, structure and function of *Neisseria* adhesins, the putative target human cell receptors, the molecular bases of their interactions and the resulting modulation of both *Neisseria* spp. and host cells in response to these interactions. Several excellent reviews cover these topics comprehensively [249,255–259]; nevertheless, we provide the reader with a brief, general discussion on conserved adhesins and other surface molecules important for initial adhesion and colonization, which may possibly help to interpret, from the view of microbiology, the extensive medical records reporting atypical infections with *Neisseria* species. In the case of atypical presentations of *Neisseria* infections in different anatomical sites, specific host cell/receptor–pathogen interactions have not been characterized; thus, an explanation for why and potentially how they occur from the view of host cell biology is still a matter of investigation.

The Type IV pilus is probably the most extensively studied *Neisseria* adhesin. Extending out from the *Neisseria* OM, pili impart twitching motility by rapid extension and retraction, facilitate uptake of foreign DNA to increase transformation frequency and are important for virulence [260]. Meningococci produce two structurally distinct types of pili, Class I and Class II. Gonococci only produce Class I pili, and both gonococcal and meningococcal Class I pili are recognized by murine monoclonal antibody SM1 [261]. Expression of pili in commensal *Neisseria* species has not been characterized as extensively as within *N. gonorrhoeae* and *N. meningitidis*, but a comparative analysis of the pilin gene in pathogenic and non-pathogenic *Neisseria* spp. demonstrated two distinct structural groups—i) the gonococcal and meningococcal Class I pilin-encoding genes and ii) the *N. lactamica*, *N. cinerea* and meningococcal Class II pilin-encoding genes [262]. Expression of pili by commensal and pathogenic *Neisseria* spp. is necessary for primary colonization of the nasopharyngeal and genitourinary niches. Pili also plays a critical role in enabling adhesive interactions of the *Neisseriae* with other anatomical niches and thus occasioning different pathologies.

The most abundant adhesion/invasion molecules embedded within the *Neisseria* OM are the Opacity-associated (Opa) and Opc proteins. The Opc protein is expressed only in *N. meningitidis* [263]. Although an *opc* pseudogene is present in *N. gonorrhoeae* and some commensal strains of *N. polysacchtaea*, significant difference was observed within the region encoding the most surface-exposed loops and there is no evidence of Opc protein expression by these organisms [263,264]. However, Opa protein is abundantly expressed and regulated in gonococci [265], meningococci [266], and the commensal strains *N. subflava*, *N. mucosa*, *N. sicca*, *N. flava*, and *N. lactamica* [267]. Other OM adhesins include the Adhesion and penetration protein (App), the Neisserial Adhesin A protein (NadA) and the *Neisseria hia/hsf* homologue NhhA protein. App is highly conserved across all *Neisseria* species, and the meningococcal App protein amino acid sequence shares ~95% and 73% identity with *N. gonorrhoeae* and *N. lactamica*, respectively [257,268,269]. The extensively characterized Trimeric Autotransporter NadA is present in ~50% of meningococcal strains but absent in *N. gonorrhoeae* and *N. lactamica* [270] and NhhA protein was reported to be expressed in *N. meningitidis* and *N. lactamica*, but not in *N. gonorrhoeae* [271].

Several other surface structures can influence bacterial attachment, e.g., CPS, LOS, and OM porin (Por) proteins. CPS expression by the meningococcus is important for virulence and capsulated and piliated meningococci are cultured from patients with sepsis and meningitis. However, CPS expression is not the only trait essential for the pathogenic potential of *N. meningitidis*. This is demonstrated by the presence of meningococcal carriage isolates expressing CPS that are not associated with disease [218–220] and by unique cases of meningococcal urethral infections with unencapsulated isolates [91] (see above, Section 3.1). Furthermore, gonococci and commensal *Neisseria* species do not express CPS and are still capable of causing infections. Similarly, there is high genetic diversity in the *ltg* loci related to the biosynthesis of LOS in pathogenic *Neisseria* and some of these genes are also found in strains considered to be non-pathogenic, e.g., *N. lactamica*, *N. subflava*, and *N. sicca*. However, *ltg* is not carried by all commensal strains [272,273]. Porins comprise up to 60% of the proteins present in the *Neisseria* OM. While most *Neisseria* species express only one Por, meningococci express two, PorA and PorB. The gonococcus is the only other *Neisseria* species known to have a *porA* pseudogene, which is silent due to frameshift and promoter mutations [274]. Phylogenetic analyses suggested an important role for horizontal genetic exchange in the emergence of different porin classes and confirmed the close evolutionary relationships of the porins from *N. meningitidis*, *N. gonorrhoeae*, *N. lactamica*, and *N. polysaccharea* [275].

The evolution of specific *Neisseria* adhesins that enable primary colonization and subsequent maintenance of a commensal carriage or progress of disease is in many respects driven by the compliant host [257]. In addition, while it might be true to state that commensal organisms and pathogens share similar adhesins, commensal *Neisseria* may not normally express the profile of virulence-associated proteins required for infection. Yet, the genetic propensity of commensal *Neisseria* species to cause disease does exist and it is reported occasionally (Table 1).

Comparative genomics of commensal human *Neisseria* species revealed that these organisms share a large repertoire of virulence-associated alleles with gonococci and meningococci, probably as a consequence of widespread virulence gene exchange amongst them [257,276,277]. A recent genome-wide analysis by Lu et al. (2019) [4] compared the genomes of 15 *N. gonorrhoeae*, 75 *N. meningitidis* and 7 commensal *Neisseria* spp. (i.e., three *N. lactamica* strains and single examples of *N. mucosa*, *N. weaveri*, *N. zoodegmatis*, and *N. elongata*) to identify genes associated with pathogenicity and niche adaptation. In this study, a core-pangenome analysis found that 452, 78, and 319 gene families were unique to gonococci, meningococci and were shared, respectively. Furthermore, abundant Simple Sequence Repeats, the molecular basis for gene phase variation, was found within these gene sets and were therefore regarded as candidates that related to their pathogenicity and ability to adapt to variable host environments [278,279]. Functional annotation analysis partly verified the relationships among them, but no certain functional information was found for at least one-third of the genes for each gene set [4].

Protein–protein interaction analysis (PPI) of unique gonococcal and meningococcal proteins found at least five and four PPI clusters in *N. gonorrhoeae* and *N. meningitidis*, respectively. These were associated mainly with basic substance transport and metabolism, genetic information processing (e.g., replication, transcription and translation), cellular processes (e.g., cell wall/membrane/envelope biogenesis and cell motility), bacteria-environment interactions (e.g., signal transduction, extracellular structures and defense mechanism), nitric oxide metabolic pathways, heme utilization and adhesion systems [4]. These proteins unique to the pathogenic *Neisseria* spp. may well be vital for their pathogenic potential and niche adaptation. Within these clusters, numerous other proteins with unknown function were also detected in the PPI analysis maps and should be investigated further for other possible interactions relevant to the pathogenicity of these species.

In this same study, commensal *Neisseria* strains showed conservation of 14 gene families and shared 39 gene families with gonococci and 11 gene families with meningococci. Interestingly, Lu et al. [4] also reported 1111 gene families that were conserved across all pathogenic and non-pathogenic *Neisseria* spp. These specific and shared genetic features could underlie the apparent differences of niche specialization and the pathogenic potential of meningococci and gonococci. They may lead us also to infer the molecular relationships between phenotypes of the 'atypical' infections with both pathogenic and 'commensal' *Neisseria* spp. Furthermore, but beyond the scope of this review, it would be worth studying the genomes of isolates from different anatomical sites, which could be partly achieved from analyzing the pubMLST.org/*Neisseria* database (Table S3). This would enable us to compare similarities between different *Neisseria* species causing the same atypical infection and the differences between the same *Neisseria* species with distinct virulence profile(s) (i.e., isolated from different anatomical sites).

7. Conclusions

In this review, we highlight the atypical infections that can be caused by pathogenic and commensal *Neisseria* spp., thereby demonstrating how effectively these organisms can colonize different anatomical niches. An increased awareness of this propensity for colonizing multiple sites would suggest a more cautious approach to diagnosing the clinical syndromes normally attributed to infection with the gonococcus or the meningococcus, and guard against dismissing as normal microbiota other *Neisseria* spp. isolated from sites other than the nasopharynx.

Supplementary Materials: The following are available online at http://www.mdpi.com/2076-0817/9/1/10/s1, Table S1: Glossary for medical terminology, Table S2: Antimicrobial treatments for atypical infections with *Neisseria* species, Table S3: The numbers of *Neisseria* species isolated from different host sites (sources), identified within the pubmlst.org/*Neisseria* database.

Author Contributions: Conceptualization, M.V.H. and M.C.; writing—original draft preparation: M.V.H. and M.C.; writing—review and editing: M.V.H. and M.C.; supervision, M.C. All authors have read and agreed to the published version of the manuscript.

Funding: This research received no external funding.

Conflicts of Interest: The authors declare no conflict of interest.

References

1. Liu, G.; Tang, C.M.; Exley, R.M. Non-pathogenic *Neisseria*: Members of an abundant, multi-habitat, diverse genus. *Microbiology* **2015**, *161*, 1297–1312. [CrossRef] [PubMed]
2. Bennet, J.S.; Bratcher, H.B.; Brehony, C.; Harrison, O.B.; Maiden, M.C.J. The genus *Neisseria*. In *Prokaryotes*; Springer: Berlin/Heidelberg, Germany, 2014; pp. 881–900.
3. Seifert, H.S. Location, Location-Commensalism, Damage and Evolution of the Pathogenic *Neisseria*. *J. Mol. Biol.* **2019**, *431*, 3010–3014. [CrossRef] [PubMed]
4. Lu, Q.F.; Cao, D.M.; Su, L.L.; Li, S.B.; Ye, G.B.; Zhu, X.Y.; Wang, J.P. Genus-Wide Comparative Genomics Analysis of *Neisseria* to Identify New Genes Associated with Pathogenicity and Niche Adaptation of *Neisseria* Pathogens. *Int. J. Genom.* **2019**, *2019*, 6015730. [CrossRef] [PubMed]
5. Neisser, A.L. Über eine der Gonorrhoe eigentümliche Micrococcusform. *Cent. Med. Wissensch* **1879**, *17*, 497–500.
6. Quillin, S.J.; Seifert, H.S. *Neisseria gonorrhoeae* host adaptation and pathogenesis. *Nat. Rev. Microbiol.* **2018**, *16*, 226–240. [CrossRef]
7. Geisler, W.M.; Yu, S.; Hook, E.W., 3rd. Chlamydial and gonococcal infection in men without polymorphonuclear leukocytes on gram stain: Implications for diagnostic approach and management. *Sex. Transm. Dis.* **2005**, *32*, 630–634. [CrossRef]
8. Jordan, S.J.; Schwebke, J.R.; Aaron, K.J.; Van Der Pol, B.; Hook, E.W., 3rd. Meatal Swabs Contain Less Cellular Material and Are Associated with a Decrease in Gram Stain Smear Quality Compared to Urethral Swabs in Men. *J. Clin. Microbiol.* **2017**, *55*, 2249–2254. [CrossRef]
9. Xiong, M.; Lan, L.; Feng, T.; Zhao, G.; Wang, F.; Hong, F.; Wu, X.; Zhang, C.; Wen, L.; Liu, A.; et al. Analysis of the sex ratio of reported gonorrhoea incidence in Shenzhen, China. *BMJ Open* **2016**, *6*, e009629. [CrossRef]
10. Stevens, J.S.; Criss, A.K. Pathogenesis of *Neisseria gonorrhoeae* in the female reproductive tract: Neutrophilic host response, sustained infection, and clinical sequelae. *Curr. Opin. Hematol.* **2018**, *25*, 13–21. [CrossRef]
11. Densen, P. Interaction of complement with *Neisseria meningitidis* and *Neisseria gonorrhoeae*. *Clin. Microbiol. Rev.* **1989**, *2*, S11–S17. [CrossRef]
12. Ngampasutadol, J.; Ram, S.; Gulati, S.; Agarwal, S.; Li, C.; Visintin, A.; Monks, B.; Madico, G.; Rice, P.A. Human factor H interacts selectively with *Neisseria gonorrhoeae* and results in species-specific complement evasion. *J. Immunol.* **2008**, *180*, 3426–3435. [CrossRef] [PubMed]

13. Sadarangani, M.; Pollard, A.J.; Gray-Owen, S.D. Opa proteins and CEACAMs: Pathways of immune engagement for pathogenic *Neisseria*. *FEMS Microbiol. Rev.* **2011**, *35*, 498–514. [CrossRef] [PubMed]
14. Evans, R.W.; Oakhill, J.S. Transferrin-mediated iron acquisition by pathogenic *Neisseria*. *Biochem. Soc. Trans.* **2002**, *30*, 705–707. [CrossRef] [PubMed]
15. Noinaj, N.; Buchanan, S.K.; Cornelissen, C.N. The transferrin-iron import system from pathogenic *Neisseria* species. *Mol. Microbiol.* **2012**, *86*, 246–257. [CrossRef] [PubMed]
16. Schoen, C.; Blom, J.; Claus, H.; Schramm-Gluck, A.; Brandt, P.; Muller, T.; Goesmann, A.; Joseph, B.; Konietzny, S.; Kurzai, O.; et al. Whole-genome comparison of disease and carriage strains provides insights into virulence evolution in *Neisseria meningitidis*. *Proc. Natl. Acad. Sci. USA* **2008**, *105*, 3473–3478. [CrossRef] [PubMed]
17. Weichselbaum, A. Über die atiologie der akuten meningitis cerebrospinalis. *Fortschritte der Medizin* **1887**, *5*, 573–583.
18. Weichselbaum, A. Über die atiologie der akuten meningitis cerebrospinalis. *Fortschritte der Medizin* **1887**, *5*, 620–626.
19. Jolley, K.A.; Wilson, D.J.; Kriz, P.; McVean, G.; Maiden, M.C. The influence of mutation, recombination, population history, and selection on patterns of genetic diversity in *Neisseria meningitidis*. *Mol. Biol. Evol.* **2005**, *22*, 562–569. [CrossRef]
20. Brandtzaeg, P.; van Deuren, M. Classification and pathogenesis of meningococcal infections. *Methods Mol. Biol.* **2012**, *799*, 21–35. [CrossRef]
21. Stephens, D.S.; Greenwood, B.; Brandtzaeg, P. Epidemic meningitis, meningococcaemia, and *Neisseria meningitidis*. *Lancet* **2007**, *369*, 2196–2210. [CrossRef]
22. Campbell, H.; Parikh, S.R.; Borrow, R.; Kaczmarski, E.; Ramsay, M.E.; Ladhani, S.N. Presentation with gastrointestinal symptoms and high case fatality associated with group W meningococcal disease (MenW) in teenagers, England, July 2015 to January 2016. *Euro Surveill.* **2016**, *21*. [CrossRef] [PubMed]
23. Carrascosa, M.F.; Casuso-Saenz, E.; Salcines-Caviedes, J.R. *Neisseria meningitidis* cellulitis. *Int. J. Infect. Dis.* **2012**, *16*, e760. [CrossRef] [PubMed]
24. Russcher, A.; Fanoy, E.; van Olden, G.D.J.; Graafland, A.D.; van der Ende, A.; Knol, M.J. Necrotising fasciitis as atypical presentation of infection with emerging *Neisseria meningitidis* serogroup W (MenW) clonal complex 11, the Netherlands, March 2017. *Euro Surveill.* **2017**, *22*, 30549. [CrossRef] [PubMed]
25. Rowley, J.; Vander Hoorn, S.; Korenromp, E.; Low, N.; Unemo, M.; Abu-Raddad, L.J.; Chico, R.M.; Smolak, A.; Newman, L.; Gottlieb, S.; et al. Chlamydia, gonorrhoea, trichomoniasis and syphilis: Global prevalence and incidence estimates, 2016. *Bull. World Health Organ.* **2019**, *97*, 548P–562P. [CrossRef] [PubMed]
26. Acevedo, R.; Bai, X.; Borrow, R.; Caugant, D.A.; Carlos, J.; Ceyhan, M.; Christensen, H.; Climent, Y.; De Wals, P.; Dinleyici, E.C.; et al. The Global Meningococcal Initiative meeting on prevention of meningococcal disease worldwide: Epidemiology, surveillance, hypervirulent strains, antibiotic resistance and high-risk populations. *Expert. Rev. Vaccines* **2019**, *18*, 15–30. [CrossRef] [PubMed]
27. Schielke, S.; Frosch, M.; Kurzai, O. Virulence determinants involved in differential host niche adaptation of *Neisseria meningitidis* and *Neisseria gonorrhoeae*. *Med. Microbiol. Immunol.* **2010**, *199*, 185–196. [CrossRef]
28. Givan, K.F.; Keyl, A. The isolation of *Neisseria* species from unusual sites. *Can. Med. Assoc. J.* **1974**, *111*, 1077–1079.
29. Gregory, J.E.; Abramson, E. Meningococci in vaginitis. *Am. J. Dis. Child.* **1971**, *121*, 423. [CrossRef]
30. Katz, A.R.; Chasnoff, R.; Komeya, A.; Lee, M.V. *Neisseria meningitidis* urethritis: A case report highlighting clinical similarities to and epidemiological differences from gonococcal urethritis. *Sex. Transm. Dis.* **2011**, *38*, 439–441. [CrossRef]
31. Lee, J.S.; Choi, H.Y.; Lee, J.E.; Lee, S.H.; Oum, B.S. Gonococcal keratoconjunctivitis in adults. *Eye (Lond.)* **2002**, *16*, 646–649. [CrossRef]
32. Odegaard, K.; Gundersen, T. Gonococcal pharyngeal infection. *Br. J. Vener. Dis.* **1973**, *49*, 350–352. [CrossRef] [PubMed]
33. Johnson, A.P. The pathogenic potential of commensal species of *Neisseria*. *J. Clin. Pathol.* **1983**, *36*, 213–223. [CrossRef] [PubMed]
34. Korting, H.C. Uncomplicated gonorrhea and disseminated gonococcal infections—Clinical aspects, diagnosis and therapy. *Urol. A* **1987**, *26*, 237–245.

35. Masi, A.T.; Eisenstein, B.I. Disseminated gonococcal infection (DGI) and gonococcal arthritis (GCA): II. Clinical manifestations, diagnosis, complications, treatment, and prevention. *Semin. Arthritis Rheum.* **1981**, *10*, 173–197. [CrossRef]
36. Bardin, T. Gonococcal arthritis. *Best Pract. Res. Clin. Rheumatol.* **2003**, *17*, 201–208. [CrossRef]
37. Rice, P.A. Gonococcal arthritis (disseminated gonococcal infection). *Infect. Dis. Clin. N. Am.* **2005**, *19*, 853–861. [CrossRef]
38. Henderson, G.; Ritchie, W.T. Gonococcal meningitis. *Rev. Neurol. Psychiatr.* **1909**, *7*, 75–87.
39. Home, E. *Practical Observations on the Treatment of Strictures in the Urethra and in the Esophagus, London*, 3rd ed.; Everard Home: London, UK, 1805; Volume 11, pp. 271–278.
40. Smith, D. Gonococcal meningitis. *Lancet* **1922**, *1*, 1217. [CrossRef]
41. Newman, A.B. The prognosis in gonococcal endocarditis. Review of literature and report of case with spontaneous recovery. *Am. Heart J.* **1933**, *8*, 821–833. [CrossRef]
42. Wall, T.C.; Peyton, R.B.; Corey, G.R. Gonococcal endocarditis: A new look at an old disease. *Medicine (Baltim.)* **1989**, *68*, 375–380. [CrossRef]
43. Thayer, W.S.; Blumer, G. Ulcerative endocarditis due to the gonococcus: Gonococcal septicemia. *Johns Hopkins Hosp. Bull.* **1896**, *7*, 57.
44. Thayer, W.S.; Lazear, J.W. A Second Case of Gonorrhoeal Septicaemia and Ulcerative Endocarditis with Observations Upon the Cardiac Complications of Gonorrhoea. *J. Exp. Med.* **1899**, *4*, 81–116. [CrossRef] [PubMed]
45. Shetty, A.; Ribeiro, D.; Evans, A.; Linnane, S. Gonococcal endocarditis: A rare complication of a common disease. *J. Clin. Pathol.* **2004**, *57*, 780–781. [CrossRef] [PubMed]
46. Schoolnik, G.K.; Buchanan, T.M.; Holmes, K.K. Gonococci causing disseminated gonococcal infection are resistant to the bactericidal action of normal human sera. *J. Clin. Investig.* **1976**, *58*, 1163–1173. [CrossRef] [PubMed]
47. Brooks, G.F.; Israel, K.S.; Petersen, B.H. Bactericidal and opsonic activity against *Neisseria gonorrhoeae* in sera from patients with disseminated gonococcal infection. *J. Infect. Dis.* **1976**, *134*, 450–462. [CrossRef] [PubMed]
48. Petersen, B.H.; Graham, J.A.; Brooks, G.F. Human deficiency of the eighth component of complement. The requirement of C8 for serum *Neisseria gonorrhoeae* bactericidal activity. *J. Clin. Investig.* **1976**, *57*, 283–290. [CrossRef]
49. Alexander, E.R. Gonorrhea in the newborn. *Ann. N. Y. Acad. Sci.* **1988**, *549*, 180–186. [CrossRef]
50. Nie, S.; Wu, Y.; Huang, L.; Pincus, D.; Tang, Y.W.; Lu, X. Gonococcal endocarditis: A case report and literature review. *Eur. J. Clin. Microbiol. Infect. Dis.* **2014**, *33*, 23–27. [CrossRef]
51. Beatrous, S.V.; Grisoli, S.B.; Riahi, R.R.; Matherne, R.J.; Matherne, R.J. Cutaneous manifestations of disseminated gonococcemia. *Dermatol. Online J.* **2017**, *23*.
52. Cowan, L. Gonococcal ulceration of the tongue in the gonococcal dermatitis syndrome. *Br. J. Vener. Dis.* **1969**, *45*, 228–231. [CrossRef]
53. Ghosn, S.H.; Kibbi, A.G. Cutaneous gonococcal infections. *Clin. Dermatol.* **2004**, *22*, 476–480. [CrossRef] [PubMed]
54. Bradford, W.L.; Kelley, H.W. Gonococcic miningitis in a new born infant with review of the literature. *Am. J. Dis. Child.* **1933**, *46*, 543–549. [CrossRef]
55. Austin, T.W.; Yang, W.; Pattison, F.M. Oropharyngeal gonorrhea: Disseminated gonococcal disease. *Can. Med. Assoc. J.* **1977**, *117*, 438. [PubMed]
56. Stolz, E.; Schuller, J. Gonococcal oro-and nasopharyngeal infection. *Br. J. Vener. Dis.* **1974**, *50*, 104–108. [CrossRef] [PubMed]
57. Yavelov, S.L.; Wiznia, A.; Brennessel, D.J.; Glaser, J.H. Disseminated gonorrhoea from a pharyngeal infection in a prepubertal child. *Int. J. Pediatr. Otorhinolaryngol.* **1984**, *7*, 297–300. [CrossRef]
58. Ratnatunga, C.S. Gonococcal pharyngitis. *Br. J. Vener. Dis.* **1972**, *48*, 184–186. [CrossRef]
59. Wiesner, P.J.; Tronca, E.; Bonin, P.; Pedersen, A.H.; Holmes, K.K. Clinical spectrum of pharyngeal gonococcal infection. *N. Engl. J. Med.* **1973**, *288*, 181–185. [CrossRef]
60. Fiumara, N.J.; Wise, H.M., Jr.; Many, M. Gonorrheal pharyngitis. *N. Engl. J. Med.* **1967**, *276*, 1248–1250. [CrossRef]
61. Schaefer, R.A.; Enzenauer, R.J.; Pruitt, A.; Corpe, R.S. Acute gonococcal flexor tenosynovitis in an adolescent male with pharyngitis. A case report and literature review. *Clin. Orthop. Relat. Res.* **1992**, *281*, 212–215.

62. Woods, C.R. Gonococcal infections in neonates and young children. *Semin. Pediatr. Infect. Dis.* **2005**, *16*, 258–270. [CrossRef]
63. Bro-Jorgensen, A.; Jensen, T. Gonococcal tonsillar infections. *Br. Med. J.* **1971**, *4*, 660–661. [CrossRef] [PubMed]
64. Diefenbach, W.C. Gonorrheal parotitis. *Oral. Surg. Oral. Med. Oral. Pathol.* **1953**, *6*, 974–975. [CrossRef]
65. Lessing, J.N.; Slingsby, T.J.; Betz, M. Hyperacute Gonococcal Keratoconjunctivitis. *J. Gen. Intern. Med.* **2019**, *34*, 477–478. [CrossRef] [PubMed]
66. Rothenberg, R. Ophthalmia neonatorum due to *Neisseria gonorrhoeae*: Prevention and treatment. *Sex. Transm. Dis.* **1979**, *6*, 187–191. [CrossRef] [PubMed]
67. Costumbrado, J.; Ghassemzadeh, S. Gonococcal Conjunctivitis. In *StatPearls*; StatPearls Publishing: Treasure Island, FL, USA, 2019.
68. Diener, B. Cesarean section complicated by gonococcal ophthalmia neonatorum. *J. Fam. Pract.* **1981**, *13*, 739–743.
69. Jacobsen, T.; Knudsen, J.D.; Weis, N.M. [Gonorrheal ophthalmia neonatorum in a premature infant delivered by cesarean section]. *Ugeskr. Laeger* **1991**, *153*, 2571. [PubMed]
70. Strand, C.L.; Arango, V.A. Gonococcal ophthalmia neonatorum after delivery by cesarean section: Report of a case. *Sex. Transm. Dis.* **1979**, *6*, 77–78. [CrossRef]
71. Belga, S.; Gratrix, J.; Smyczek, P.; Bertholet, L.; Read, R.; Roelofs, K.; Singh, A.E. Gonococcal Conjunctivitis in Adults: Case Report and Retrospective Review of Cases in Alberta, Canada, 2000–2016. *Sex. Transm. Dis.* **2019**, *46*, 47–51. [CrossRef]
72. McAnena, L.; Knowles, S.J.; Curry, A.; Cassidy, L. Prevalence of gonococcal conjunctivitis in adults and neonates. *Eye (Lond.)* **2015**, *29*, 875–880. [CrossRef]
73. Varady, E.; Nsanze, H.; Slattery, T. Gonococcal scalp abscess in a neonate delivered by caesarean section. *Sex. Transm. Infect.* **1998**, *74*, 451. [CrossRef]
74. Bodsworth, N.J.; Price, R.; Nelson, M.J. A case of gonococcal mastitis in a male. *Genitourin. Med.* **1993**, *69*, 222–223. [CrossRef] [PubMed]
75. Ceniceros, A.; Galen, B.; Madaline, T. Gonococcal breast abscess. *IDCases* **2019**, *18*, e00620. [CrossRef] [PubMed]
76. Bateman, A.C. Unusual cause of a wound infection. *J. Appl. Lab. Med.* **2017**, *2*, 444–448. [CrossRef]
77. Pendle, S.; Barnes, T. *Neisseria gonorrhoeae* isolated from an unexpected site. *Sex. Health* **2016**, *13*, 593–594. [CrossRef]
78. Lewis, J.F.; Alexander, J.J. Isolation of *Neisseria meningitidis* from the vagina and cervix. *Am. J. Clin. Pathol.* **1974**, *61*, 216–217. [CrossRef]
79. Jones, R.N.; Slepack, J.; Eades, A. Fatal neonatal meningococcal meningitis. Association with maternal cervical-vaginal colonization. *JAMA* **1976**, *236*, 2652–2653. [CrossRef]
80. Sunderland, W.A.; Harris, H.H.; Spence, D.A.; Lawson, H.W. Meningococcemia in a newborn infant whose mother had meningococcal vaginitis. *J. Pediatr.* **1972**, *81*, 856. [CrossRef]
81. Chacon-Cruz, E.; Alvelais-Palacios, J.A.; Rodriguez-Valencia, J.A.; Lopatynsky-Reyes, E.Z.; Volker-Soberanes, M.L.; Rivas-Landeros, R.M. Meningococcal Neonatal Purulent Conjunctivitis/Sepsis and Asymptomatic Carriage of *N. meningitidis* in Mother's Vagina and Both Parents' Nasopharynx. *Case Rep. Infect. Dis.* **2017**, *2017*, 6132857. [CrossRef]
82. Murray, E.G.D. Meningococcus infections of the male urogenital tract and the liability to confusion with gonococcus. *Urol Cutan. Rev.* **1939**, *43*, 739–741.
83. Givan, K.F.; Thomas, B.W.; Johnston, A.G. Isolation of *Neisseria meningitidis* from the urethra, cervix, and anal canal: Further observations. *Br. J. Vener. Dis.* **1977**, *53*, 109–112. [CrossRef]
84. Volk, J.; Kraus, S.J. Asymptomatic meningococcal urethritis. Possible protective value against gonococcal infection by bacteriocin production. *Br. J. Vener. Dis.* **1973**, *49*, 511–512. [CrossRef] [PubMed]
85. Carpenter, C.M.; Charles, R. Isolation of Meningococcus from the Genitourinary Tract of Seven Patients. *Am. J. Public Health Nations Health* **1942**, *32*, 640–643. [CrossRef] [PubMed]
86. Faur, Y.C.; Wilson, M.E.; May, P.S. Isolation of *N. meningitidis* from patients in a gonorrhea screen program: A four-year survey in New York City. *Am. J. Public Health* **1981**, *71*, 53–58. [CrossRef] [PubMed]
87. Kanemitsu, N.; Hayashi, I.; Satoh, N.; Hayakawa, T.; Mitsuya, H.; Hayase, Y.; Hiramoto, K.; Kojima, M. Acute urethritis caused by *Neisseria meningitidis*. *Int. J. Urol.* **2003**, *10*, 346–347. [CrossRef] [PubMed]

88. Harrison, O.B.; Cole, K.; Peters, J.; Cresswell, F.; Dean, G.; Eyre, D.W.; Paul, J.; Maiden, M.C. Genomic analysis of urogenital and rectal *Neisseria meningitidis* isolates reveals encapsulated hyperinvasive meningococci and coincident multidrug-resistant gonococci. *Sex. Transm. Infect.* **2017**, *93*, 445–451. [CrossRef] [PubMed]
89. Winterscheid, K.K.; Whittington, W.L.; Roberts, M.C.; Schwebke, J.R.; Holmes, K.K. Decreased susceptibility to penicillin G and Tet M plasmids in genital and anorectal isolates of *Neisseria meningitidis*. *Antimicrob. Agents Chemother.* **1994**, *38*, 1661–1663. [CrossRef]
90. Retchless, A.C.; Kretz, C.B.; Chang, H.Y.; Bazan, J.A.; Abrams, A.J.; Norris Turner, A.; Jenkins, L.T.; Trees, D.L.; Tzeng, Y.L.; Stephens, D.S.; et al. Expansion of a urethritis-associated *Neisseria meningitidis* clade in the United States with concurrent acquisition of *N. gonorrhoeae* alleles. *BMC Genom.* **2018**, *19*, 176. [CrossRef]
91. Bazan, J.A.; Turner, A.N.; Kirkcaldy, R.D.; Retchless, A.C.; Kretz, C.B.; Briere, E.; Tzeng, Y.L.; Stephens, D.S.; Maierhofer, C.; Del Rio, C.; et al. Large Cluster of *Neisseria meningitidis* Urethritis in Columbus, Ohio, 2015. *Clin. Infect. Dis.* **2017**, *65*, 92–99. [CrossRef]
92. Tzeng, Y.L.; Bazan, J.A.; Turner, A.N.; Wang, X.; Retchless, A.C.; Read, T.D.; Toh, E.; Nelson, D.E.; Del Rio, C.; Stephens, D.S. Emergence of a new *Neisseria meningitidis* clonal complex 11 lineage 11.2 clade as an effective urogenital pathogen. *Proc. Natl. Acad. Sci. USA* **2017**, *114*, 4237–4242. [CrossRef]
93. Hagman, M.; Forslin, L.; Moi, H.; Danielsson, D. *Neisseria meningitidis* in specimens from urogenital sites. Is increased awareness necessary? *Sex. Transm. Dis.* **1991**, *18*, 228–232. [CrossRef]
94. Wilson, A.P.; Wolff, J.; Atia, W. Acute urethritis due to *Neisseria meningitidis* group A acquired by orogenital contact: Case report. *Genitourin. Med.* **1989**, *65*, 122–123. [CrossRef] [PubMed]
95. Keys, T.F.; Hecht, R.H.; Chow, A.W. Endocervical *Neisseria meningitidis* with meningococcemia. *N. Engl. J. Med.* **1971**, *285*, 505–506. [CrossRef] [PubMed]
96. Harriau, P.; Ramanantsoa, C.; Pierre, F.; Riou, J.Y.; Quentin, R. Endocervical infection in a pregnant woman caused by *Neisseria meningitidis*: Evidence of associated oropharyngeal colonization of the male partner. *Eur. J. Obstet. Gynecol. Reprod. Biol.* **1997**, *74*, 145–147. [CrossRef]
97. Fiorito, S.M.; Galarza, P.G.; Sparo, M.; Pagano, E.I.; Oviedo, C.I. An unusual transmission of *Neisseria meningitidis*: Neonatal conjunctivitis acquired at delivery from the mother's endocervical infection. *Sex. Transm. Dis.* **2001**, *28*, 29–32. [CrossRef]
98. Mitchell, S.R.; Katz, P. Disseminated neisserial infection in pregnancy: The empress may have a change of clothing. *Obstet. Gynecol. Surv.* **1989**, *44*, 780–788.
99. Bhutta, Z.A.; Khan, I.A.; Agha, Z. Fatal intrauterine meningococcal infection. *Pediatr. Infect. Dis. J.* **1991**, *10*, 868–869.
100. Irani, F.; Ruddell, T. Meningococcal conjunctivitis. *Aust. N. Z. J. Ophthalmol.* **1997**, *25*, 167–168. [CrossRef]
101. Unal Yilmaz, G.; Alkan, M.; Vatansever Ozbek, U.; Tugrul, H.M. [Healthcare-associated *Neisseria meningitidis* W135 conjunctivitis]. *Mikrobiyol. Bul.* **2013**, *47*, 722–726. [CrossRef]
102. Moraga Llop, F.A.; Barquet Esteve, N.; Domingo Pedrol, P.; Gallart Catala, A. [Primary meningococcal conjunctivitis: Implications beyond the conjunctiva]. *Med. Clin. (Barc)* **1996**, *107*, 130–132.
103. Barquet, N.; Gasser, I.; Domingo, P.; Moraga, F.A.; Macaya, A.; Elcuaz, R. Primary meningococcal conjunctivitis: Report of 21 patients and review. *Rev. Infect. Dis.* **1990**, *12*, 838–847. [CrossRef]
104. Holmberg, L.; Moestrup, T. Meningitis following conjunctivitis. *J. Pediatr.* **1979**, *94*, 339. [CrossRef]
105. Nussbaum, E.; Jeyaranjan, T.; Feldman, F. Primary meningococcal conjunctivitis followed by meningitis. *J. Pediatr.* **1978**, *92*, 784–785. [CrossRef]
106. Dryden, A.W.; Rana, M.; Pandey, P. Primary meningococcal conjunctivitis: An unusual case of transmission by saliva. *Digit. J. Ophthalmol.* **2016**, *22*, 25–27. [CrossRef] [PubMed]
107. Holdsworth, G.; Jackson, H.; Kaczmarski, E. Meningococcal infection from saliva. *Lancet* **1996**, *348*, 1443. [CrossRef]
108. Hansman, D. Neonatal meningococcal conjunctivitis. *Br. Med. J.* **1972**, *1*, 748. [CrossRef] [PubMed]
109. Poulos, R.G.; Smedley, E.J.; Ferson, M.J.; Bolisetty, S.; Tapsall, J.W. Refining the public health response to primary meningococcal conjunctivitis. *Commun. Dis. Intell. Q Rep.* **2002**, *26*, 592–595.
110. de Souza, A.L.; Seguro, A.C. Conjunctivitis secondary to *Neisseria meningitidis*: A potential vertical transmission pathway. *Clin. Pediatr. (Phila.)* **2009**, *48*, 119. [CrossRef]
111. Ellis, M.; Weindling, A.M.; Davidson, D.C.; Ho, N.; Damjanovic, V. Neonatal meningococcal conjunctivitis associated with meningococcal meningitis. *Arch. Dis. Child.* **1992**, *67*, 1219–1220. [CrossRef]

112. Agrawal, P.; Yellachich, D.; Kirkpatrick, N. Retinal detachment following meningococcal endophthalmitis. *Eye (Lond.)* **2007**, *21*, 450–451. [CrossRef]
113. Chacko, E.; Filtcroft, I.; Condon, P.I. Meningococcal septicemia presenting as bilateral endophthalmitis. *J. Cataract. Refract. Surg.* **2005**, *31*, 432–434. [CrossRef]
114. Balaskas, K.; Potamitou, D. Endogenous endophthalmitis secondary to bacterial meningitis from *Neisseria Meningitidis*: A case report and review of the literature. *Cases J.* **2009**, *2*, 149. [CrossRef] [PubMed]
115. Barnard, T.; Das, A.; Hickey, S. Bilateral endophthalmitis as an initial presentation in meningococcal meningitis. *Arch. Ophthalmol.* **1997**, *115*, 1472–1473. [CrossRef] [PubMed]
116. Chhabra, M.S.; Noble, A.G.; Kumar, A.V.; Mets, M.B. *Neisseria meningitidis* endogenous endophthalmitis presenting as anterior uveitis. *J. Pediatr. Ophthalmol. Strabismus* **2007**, *44*, 309–310. [PubMed]
117. Sleep, T.; Graham, M. A case of meningococcal endophthalmitis in a well patient. *Br. J. Ophthalmol.* **1997**, *81*, 1016–1017. [CrossRef] [PubMed]
118. Kerkhoff, F.T.; van der Zee, A.; Bergmans, A.M.; Rothova, A. Polymerase chain reaction detection of *Neisseria meningitidis* in the intraocular fluid of a patient with endogenous endophthalmitis but without associated meningitis. *Ophthalmology* **2003**, *110*, 2134–2136. [CrossRef]
119. Kallinich, T.; von Bernuth, H.; Kuhns, M.; Elias, J.; Bertelmann, E.; Pleyer, U. Fulminant Endophthalmitis in a Child Caused by *Neisseria meningitidis* Serogroup C Detected by Specific DNA. *J. Pediatric Infect. Dis. Soc.* **2016**, *5*, e13–e16. [CrossRef]
120. Yusuf, I.H.; Sipkova, Z.; Patel, S.; Benjamin, L. *Neisseria meningitidis* endogenous endophthalmitis with meningitis in an immunocompetent child. *Ocul. Immunol. Inflamm.* **2014**, *22*, 398–402. [CrossRef]
121. Gartaganis, S.P.; Eliopoulou, M.J.; Georgakopoulos, C.D.; Koliopoulos, J.X.; Mela, E.K. Bilateral panophthalmitis as the initial presentation of meningococcal meningitis in an infant. *J. AAPOS* **2001**, *5*, 260–261. [CrossRef]
122. Abandeh, F.I.; Balada-Llasat, J.M.; Pancholi, P.; Risaliti, C.M.; Maher, W.E.; Bazan, J.A. A rare case of *Neisseria bacilliformis* native valve endocarditis. *Diagn. Microbiol. Infect. Dis.* **2012**, *73*, 378–379. [CrossRef]
123. Masliah-Planchon, J.; Breton, G.; Jarlier, V.; Simon, A.; Benveniste, O.; Herson, S.; Drieux, L. Endocarditis due to *Neisseria bacilliformis* in a patient with a bicuspid aortic valve. *J. Clin. Microbiol.* **2009**, *47*, 1973–1975. [CrossRef]
124. Han, X.Y.; Hong, T.; Falsen, E. *Neisseria bacilliformis* sp. nov. isolated from human infections. *J. Clin. Microbiol.* **2006**, *44*, 474–479. [CrossRef] [PubMed]
125. Allison, K.; Clarridge, J.E., 3rd. Long-term respiratory tract infection with canine-associated *Pasteurella dagmatis* and *Neisseria canis* in a patient with chronic bronchiectasis. *J. Clin. Microbiol.* **2005**, *43*, 4272–4274. [CrossRef] [PubMed]
126. Safton, S.; Cooper, G.; Harrison, M.; Wright, L.; Walsh, P. *Neisseria canis* infection: A case report. *Commun. Dis. Intell.* **1999**, *23*, 221. [PubMed]
127. Southern, P.M., Jr.; Kutscher, A.E. Bacteremia due to *Neisseria cinerea*: Report of two cases. *Diagn. Microbiol. Infect. Dis.* **1987**, *7*, 143–147. [CrossRef]
128. Kirchgesner, V.; Plesiat, P.; Dupont, M.J.; Estavoyer, J.M.; Guibourdenche, M.; Riou, J.Y.; Michel-Briand, Y. Meningitis and septicemia due to *Neisseria cinerea*. *Clin. Infect. Dis.* **1995**, *21*, 1351. [CrossRef] [PubMed]
129. Wang, D.N.; Luo, Z.H.; Wang, H. [Diagnosis and treatment of genitourinary infection with non-gonococcal *Neisseria* in men]. *Zhonghua Nan Ke Xue* **2009**, *15*, 499–504. [PubMed]
130. Garcia, S.D.; Descole, E.M.; Famiglietti, A.M.; Lopez, E.G.; Vay, C.A. Infection of the urinary tract caused by *Neisseria cinerea*. *Enferm. Infecc. Microbiol. Clin.* **1996**, *14*, 576.
131. Taegtmeyer, M.; Saxena, R.; Corkill, J.E.; Anijeet, H.; Parry, C.M. Ciprofloxacin treatment of bacterial peritonitis associated with chronic ambulatory peritoneal dialysis caused by *Neisseria cinerea*. *J. Clin. Microbiol.* **2006**, *44*, 3040–3041. [CrossRef]
132. Bourbeau, P.; Holla, V.; Piemontese, S. Ophthalmia neonatorum caused by *Neisseria cinerea*. *J. Clin. Microbiol.* **1990**, *28*, 1640–1641.
133. Fiorito, T.M.; Noor, A.; Silletti, R.; Krilov, L.R. Neonatal Conjunctivitis Caused by *Neisseria cinerea*: A Case of Mistaken Identity. *J. Pediatric. Infect. Dis. Soc.* **2018**, *8*, 478–480. [CrossRef]
134. Wroblewski, D.; Cole, J.; McGinnis, J.; Perez, M.; Wilson, H.; Mingle, L.A.; Musser, K.A.; Wolfgang, W.J. *Neisseria dumasiana* sp. nov. from human sputum and a dog's mouth. *Int. J. Syst. Evol. Microbiol.* **2017**, *67*, 4304–4310. [CrossRef] [PubMed]

135. Grant, P.E.; Brenner, D.J.; Steigerwalt, A.G.; Hollis, D.G.; Weaver, R.E. *Neisseria elongata* subsp. *nitroreducens* subsp. nov., formerly CDC group M-6, a gram-negative bacterium associated with endocarditis. *J. Clin. Microbiol.* **1990**, *28*, 2591–2596. [PubMed]
136. Samannodi, M.; Vakkalanka, S.; Zhao, A.; Hocko, M. *Neisseria elongata* endocarditis of a native aortic valve. *BMJ Case Rep.* **2016**, *2016*. [CrossRef]
137. Hofstad, T.; Hope, O.; Falsen, E. Septicaemia with *Neisseria elongata* ssp. *nitroreducens* in a patient with hypertrophic obstructive cardiomyopathia. *Scand. J. Infect. Dis.* **1998**, *30*, 200–201. [CrossRef] [PubMed]
138. Garner, J.; Briant, R.H. Osteomyelitis caused by a bacterium known as M6. *J. Infect.* **1986**, *13*, 298–300. [CrossRef]
139. Scott, R.M. Bacterial endocarditis due to *Neisseria flava*. *J. Pediatr.* **1971**, *78*, 673–675. [CrossRef]
140. Matlage, W.T.; Harrison, P.E.; Greene, J.A. *Neisseria flava* endocarditis; with report of a case. *Ann. Intern. Med.* **1950**, *33*, 1494–1498. [CrossRef]
141. Sinave, C.P.; Ratzan, K.R. Infective endocarditis caused by *Neisseria flavescens*. *Am. J. Med.* **1987**, *82*, 163–164. [CrossRef]
142. Szabo, S.; Lieberman, J.P.; Lue, Y.A. Unusual pathogens in narcotic-associated endocarditis. *Rev. Infect. Dis.* **1990**, *12*, 412–415. [CrossRef]
143. Branham, S.E. A new meningococcus-like organism (*Neisseria flavescens* nsp) from epidemic meningitis. *Public Health Rep.* **1930**, *45*, 845–849. [CrossRef]
144. Prentice, A.W. *Neisseria flavescens* as a cause of meningitis. *Lancet* **1957**, *272*, 613–614. [CrossRef]
145. Feder, H.M., Jr.; Garibaldi, R.A. The significance of nongonococcal, nonmeningococcal *Neisseria* isolates from blood cultures. *Rev. Infect. Dis.* **1984**, *6*, 181–188. [CrossRef] [PubMed]
146. Wertlake, P.T.; Williams, T.W., Jr. Septicaemia caused by *Neisseria flavescens*. *J. Clin. Pathol.* **1968**, *21*, 437–439. [CrossRef] [PubMed]
147. Huang, L.; Ma, L.; Fan, K.; Li, Y.; Xie, L.; Xia, W.; Gu, B.; Liu, G. Necrotizing pneumonia and empyema caused by *Neisseria flavescens* infection. *J. Thorac. Dis.* **2014**, *6*, 553–557. [CrossRef]
148. Wax, L. The identity of *Neisseria* other than the gonococcus isolated from the genito-urinary tract. *J. Vener. Dis. Infect.* **1950**, *31*, 208–213.
149. Denning, D.W.; Gill, S.S. *Neisseria lactamica* meningitis following skull trauma. *Rev. Infect. Dis.* **1991**, *13*, 216–218. [CrossRef]
150. Lauer, B.A.; Fisher, C.E. *Neisseria lactamica* meningitis. *Am. J. Dis. Child.* **1976**, *130*, 198–199. [CrossRef]
151. Wilson, H.D.; Overman, T.L. Septicemia due to *Neisseria lactamica*. *J. Clin. Microbiol.* **1976**, *4*, 214–215.
152. Fisher, L.S.; Edelstein, P.; Guze, L.B. Letter: *Neisseria lactamicus* pharyngitis. *JAMA* **1975**, *233*, 22. [CrossRef]
153. Zavascki, A.P.; Fritscher, L.; Superti, S.; Dias, C.; Kroth, L.; Traesel, M.A.; Antonello, I.C.; Saitovitch, D. First case report of *Neisseria lactamica* causing cavitary lung disease in an adult organ transplant recipient. *J. Clin. Microbiol.* **2006**, *44*, 2666–2668. [CrossRef]
154. Wang, C.Y.; Chuang, Y.M.; Teng, L.J.; Lee, L.N.; Yang, P.C.; Kuo, S.H.; Hsueh, P.R. Bacteraemic pneumonia caused by *Neisseria lactamica* with reduced susceptibility to penicillin and ciprofloxacin in an adult with liver cirrhosis. *J. Med. Microbiol.* **2006**, *55*, 1151–1152. [CrossRef] [PubMed]
155. Jephcott, A.E.; Morton, R.S. Isolation of *Neisseria lactamicus* from a genital site. *Lancet* **1972**, *2*, 739–740. [CrossRef]
156. Brunton, W.A.T.; Young, H.; Fraser, D.R.K. Isolation of *Neisseria lactamica* from the female genital tract. *Br. J. Vener. Dis.* **1980**, *56*, 325–326.
157. Brodie, E.; Adler, J.L.; Daly, A.K. Bacterial endocarditis due to an unusual species of encapsulated *Neisseria*. *Neisseria mucosa* endocarditis. *Am. J. Dis. Child.* **1971**, *122*, 433–437. [CrossRef]
158. Pilmis, B.; Lefort, A.; Lecuit, M.; Join-Lambert, O.; Nassif, X.; Lortholary, O.; Charlier, C. Endocarditis due to *Neisseria mucosa*: Case report and review of 21 cases: A rare and severe cause of endocarditis. *J. Infect.* **2014**, *68*, 601–604. [CrossRef]
159. Ingram, R.J.; Cornere, B.; Ellis-Pegler, R.B. Endocarditis due to *Neisseria mucosa*: Two case reports and review. *Clin. Infect. Dis.* **1992**, *15*, 321–324. [CrossRef]
160. Sirot, J.; Cluzel, M. "*Neisseria mucosa*" responsible for purulent meningitis of children. *Ann. Inst. Pasteur. (Paris)* **1972**, *122*, 53–61.
161. Stotka, J.L.; Rupp, M.E.; Meier, F.A.; Markowitz, S.M. Meningitis due to *Neisseria mucosa*: Case report and review. *Rev. Infect. Dis.* **1991**, *13*, 837–841. [CrossRef]

162. Locy, C.J. Neisseria mucosa septicemia. *Clin. Microbiol. Newsl.* **1995**, *17*, 72. [CrossRef]
163. Thorsteinsson, S.B.; Minuth, J.N.; Musher, D.M. Postpneumonectomy empyema due to *Neisseria mucosa*. *Am. J. Clin. Pathol.* **1975**, *64*, 534–536. [CrossRef]
164. Hanau-Bercot, B.; Rottman, M.; Raskine, L.; Jacob, D.; Barnaud, G.; Gabarre, A.; Sanson Le Pors, M.J. Clinical resistance to amoxicillin of a gravidic urinary tract infection caused by *Neisseria mucosa*. *J. Infect.* **2001**, *43*, 160–161. [CrossRef] [PubMed]
165. Washburn, R.G.; Bryan, C.S.; DiSalvo, A.F.; Macher, A.M.; Gallin, J.I. Visceral botryomycosis caused by *Neisseria mucosa* in a patient with chronic granulomatous disease. *J. Infect. Dis.* **1985**, *151*, 563–564. [CrossRef] [PubMed]
166. Abiteboul, M.; Mazieres, B.; Causse, B.; Moatti, N.; Arlet, J. Septic arthritis of the knee due to *Neisseria mucosa*. *Clin. Rheumatol.* **1985**, *4*, 83–85. [CrossRef] [PubMed]
167. Van Linthoudt, D.; Modde, H.; Ott, H. *Neisseria mucosa* septic arthritis. *Br. J. Rheumatol.* **1987**, *26*, 314. [CrossRef]
168. Alamri, Y.; Keene, A.; Pithie, A. Acute Cystitis Caused by Commensal *Neisseria oralis*: A Case Report and Review of the Literature. *Infect. Disord. Drug Targets* **2017**, *17*, 64–66. [CrossRef]
169. Wolfgang, W.J.; Passaretti, T.V.; Jose, R.; Cole, J.; Coorevits, A.; Carpenter, A.N.; Jose, S.; Van Landschoot, A.; Izard, J.; Kohlerschmidt, D.J.; et al. *Neisseria oralis* sp. nov., isolated from healthy gingival plaque and clinical samples. *Int. J. Syst. Evol. Microbiol.* **2013**, *63*, 1323–1328. [CrossRef]
170. Breslin, A.B.; Biggs, J.C.; Hall, G.V. Bacterial endocarditis due to *Neisseria perflava* in a patient hypersensitive to penicillin. *Australas. Ann. Med.* **1967**, *16*, 245–249. [CrossRef]
171. Clark, H.; Patton, R.D. Postcardiotomy endocarditis due to *Neisseria perflava* on a prosthetic aortic valve. *Ann. Intern. Med.* **1968**, *68*, 386–389. [CrossRef]
172. Wolfgang, W.J.; Carpenter, A.N.; Cole, J.A.; Gronow, S.; Habura, A.; Jose, S.; Nazarian, E.J.; Kohlerschmidt, D.J.; Limberger, R.; Schoonmaker-Bopp, D.; et al. *Neisseria wadsworthii* sp. nov. and *Neisseria shayeganii* sp. nov., isolated from clinical specimens. *Int. J. Syst. Evol. Microbiol.* **2011**, *61*, 91–98. [CrossRef]
173. Schultz, O.T. Acute vegetative endocarditis with multiple secondary foci involvement due to *Micrococcus pharyngitidis-siccae*. *JAMA* **1918**, *71*, 1739–1741. [CrossRef]
174. Graef, I.; de la Chapelle, C.E.; Vance, M.C. *Micrococcus pharyngis siccus* endocarditis. *Am. J. Pathol.* **1932**, *8*, 341, 347–354. [PubMed]
175. Kirlew, C.; Wilmot, K.; Salinas, J.L. *Neisseria sicca* Endocarditis Presenting as Multiple Embolic Brain Infarcts. *Open Forum Infect. Dis.* **2015**, *2*, ofv105. [CrossRef] [PubMed]
176. Sommerstein, R.; Ramsay, D.; Dubuis, O.; Waser, S.; Aebersold, F.; Vogt, M. Fatal *Neisseria sicca* endocarditis. *Infection* **2013**, *41*, 747–749. [CrossRef] [PubMed]
177. Bansmer, C.; Brem, J. Acute meningitis caused by *Neisseria sicca*. *N. Engl. J. Med.* **1948**, *238*, 596. [CrossRef]
178. Carter, J.E.; Mizell, K.N.; Evans, T.N. *Neisseria sicca* meningitis following intracranial hemorrhage and ventriculostomy tube placement. *Clin. Neurol. Neurosurg.* **2007**, *109*, 918–921. [CrossRef] [PubMed]
179. Alcid, D.V. *Neisseria sicca* pneumonia. *Chest* **1980**, *77*, 123–124. [CrossRef]
180. Wilkinson, A.E. Occurrence of *Neisseria* other than the gonococcus in the genital tract. *Br. J. Vener. Dis.* **1952**, *28*, 24–27. [CrossRef]
181. Weaver, J.D. Nongonorrheal vulvovaginitis due to gram-negative intracellular diplococci. *Am. J. Obstet. Gynecol.* **1950**, *60*, 257–260. [CrossRef]
182. Gomez-Camarasa, C.; Liebana-Martos, C.; Navarro-Mari, J.M.; Gutierrez-Fernandez, J. Detection of unusual uropathogens during a period of three years in a regional hospital. *Rev. Esp Quimioter.* **2015**, *28*, 86–91.
183. Connaughton, F.W.; Rountree, P.M. A fatal case of infective endocarditis due to *Neisseria flava*. *Med. J. Aust.* **1939**, *2*, 138–139. [CrossRef]
184. Flores, J.; Lloret, A.; Bellver, F.; Segarra, C.; Monzo, E. [Infectious endocarditis by *Neisseria subflava* in two HIV drug users]. *An. Med. Interna* **1997**, *14*, 267–268. [PubMed]
185. Benson, H.; Brennwasser, R.; D'andrea, D. *Neisseria subflava* (Bergey) meningitis in an infant. *J. Infect. Dis.* **1928**, *43*, 516–524. [CrossRef]
186. Lewin, R.A.; Hughes, W.T. *Neisseria subflava* as a cause of meningitis and septicemia in children. Report of five cases. *JAMA* **1966**, *195*, 821–823. [CrossRef]
187. Wakui, D.; Nagashima, G.; Otsuka, Y.; Takada, T.; Ueda, T.; Tanaka, Y.; Hashimoto, T. A case of meningitis due to *Neisseria subflava* after ventriculostomy. *J. Infect. Chemother.* **2012**, *18*, 115–118. [CrossRef] [PubMed]

188. Carpenter, C.M. Isolation of *Neisseria flava* from the Genitourinary Tract of Three Patients. *Am. J. Public Health Nations Health* **1943**, *33*, 135–136. [CrossRef] [PubMed]
189. Janda, W.M.; Senseng, C.; Todd, K.M.; Schreckenberger, P.C. Asymptomatic *Neisseria subflava* biovar perflava bacteriuria in a child with obstructive uropathy. *Eur. J. Clin. Microbiol. Infect. Dis.* **1993**, *12*, 540–545. [CrossRef] [PubMed]
190. Carlson, P.; Kontiainen, S.; Anttila, P.; Eerola, E. Septicemia caused by *Neisseria weaveri*. *Clin. Infect. Dis.* **1997**, *24*, 739. [CrossRef]
191. Panagea, S.; Bijoux, R.; Corkill, J.E.; Al Rashidi, F.; Hart, C.A. A case of lower respiratory tract infection caused by *Neisseria weaveri* and review of the literature. *J. Infect.* **2002**, *44*, 96–98. [CrossRef]
192. Kocyigit, I.; Unal, A.; Sipahioglu, M.; Tokgoz, B.; Oymak, O.; Utas, C. Peritoneal dialysis-related peritonitis due to *Neisseria weaveri*: The first case report. *Perit. Dial. Int.* **2010**, *30*, 116–117. [CrossRef]
193. Andersen, B.M.; Steigerwalt, A.G.; O'Connor, S.P.; Hollis, D.G.; Weyant, R.S.; Weaver, R.E.; Brenner, D.J. *Neisseria weaveri* sp. nov., formerly CDC group M-5, a gram-negative bacterium associated with dog bite wounds. *J. Clin. Microbiol.* **1993**, *31*, 2456–2466.
194. Holmes, B.; Costas, M.; On, S.L.; Vandamme, P.; Falsen, E.; Kersters, K. *Neisseria weaveri* sp. nov. (formerly CDC group M-5), from dog bite wounds of humans. *Int. J. Syst. Bacteriol.* **1993**, *43*, 687–693. [CrossRef] [PubMed]
195. Grob, J.J.; Bollet, C.; Richard, M.A.; De Micco, P.; Bonerandi, J.J. Extensive skin ulceration due to EF-4 bacterial infection in a patient with AIDS. *Br. J. Dermatol.* **1989**, *121*, 507–510. [CrossRef] [PubMed]
196. Catlin, B.W. *Branhamella catarrhalis*: An organism gaining respect as a pathogen. *Clin. Microbiol. Rev.* **1990**, *3*, 293–320. [CrossRef] [PubMed]
197. Pettersson, B.; Kodjo, A.; Ronaghi, M.; Uhlen, M.; Tonjum, T. Phylogeny of the family Moraxellaceae by 16S rDNA sequence analysis, with special emphasis on differentiation of *Moraxella* species. *Int. J. Syst. Bacteriol.* **1998**, *48*, 75–89. [CrossRef]
198. Dillard, J.P.; Seifert, H.S. A variable genetic island specific for *Neisseria gonorrhoeae* is involved in providing DNA for natural transformation and is found more often in disseminated infection isolates. *Mol. Microbiol.* **2001**, *41*, 263–277. [CrossRef]
199. Dillard, J.P.; Seifert, H.S. A peptidoglycan hydrolase similar to bacteriophage endolysins acts as an autolysin in *Neisseria gonorrhoeae*. *Mol. Microbiol.* **1997**, *25*, 893–901. [CrossRef]
200. Frazer, A.D.; Menton, J. Gonococcal Stomatitis. *Br. Med. J.* **1931**, *1*, 1020–1022. [CrossRef]
201. Copping, A.A. Stomatitis caused by gonococcus. *J. Am. Dent. Assoc.* **1954**, *49*, 567.
202. Schmidt, H.; Hjorting-Hansen, E.; Philipsen, H.P. Gonococcal stomatitis. *Acta Derm. Venereol.* **1961**, *41*, 324–327.
203. Escobar, V.; Farman, A.G.; Arm, R.N. Oral gonococcal infection. *Int. J. Oral. Surg.* **1984**, *13*, 549–554. [CrossRef]
204. Kohn, S.R.; Shaffer, J.F.; Chomenko, A.G. Primary gonococcal stomatitis. *JAMA* **1972**, *219*, 86. [CrossRef] [PubMed]
205. Regan, D.G.; Hui, B.B.; Wood, J.G.; Fifer, H.; Lahra, M.M.; Whiley, D.M. Treatment for pharyngeal gonorrhoea under threat. *Lancet Infect. Dis.* **2018**, *18*, 1175–1177. [CrossRef]
206. Fifer, H.; Natarajan, U.; Jones, L.; Alexander, S.; Hughes, G.; Golparian, D.; Unemo, M. Failure of Dual Antimicrobial Therapy in Treatment of Gonorrhea. *N. Engl. J. Med.* **2016**, *374*, 2504–2506. [CrossRef] [PubMed]
207. Eyre, D.W.; Sanderson, N.D.; Lord, E.; Regisford-Reimmer, N.; Chau, K.; Barker, L.; Morgan, M.; Newnham, R.; Golparian, D.; Unemo, M.; et al. Gonorrhoea treatment failure caused by a *Neisseria gonorrhoeae* strain with combined ceftriaxone and high-level azithromycin resistance, England, February 2018. *Euro Surveill.* **2018**, *23*, 1800323. [CrossRef] [PubMed]
208. Leibowitz, H.M. The red eye. *N. Engl. J. Med.* **2000**, *343*, 345–351. [CrossRef]
209. Moi, H.; Blee, K.; Horner, P.J. Management of non-gonococcal urethritis. *BMC Infect. Dis.* **2015**, *15*, 294. [CrossRef]
210. Kroll, J.S.; Wilks, K.E.; Farrant, J.L.; Langford, P.R. Natural genetic exchange between *Haemophilus* and *Neisseria*: Intergeneric transfer of chromosomal genes between major human pathogens. *Proc. Natl. Acad. Sci. USA* **1998**, *95*, 12381–12385. [CrossRef]

211. Tzeng, Y.L.; Thomas, J.; Stephens, D.S. Regulation of capsule in *Neisseria meningitidis*. *Crit. Rev. Microbiol.* **2016**, *42*, 759–772. [CrossRef]
212. Hammerschmidt, S.; Birkholz, C.; Zahringer, U.; Robertson, B.D.; van Putten, J.; Ebeling, O.; Frosch, M. Contribution of genes from the capsule gene complex (*cps*) to lipooligosaccharide biosynthesis and serum resistance in *Neisseria meningitidis*. *Mol. Microbiol.* **1994**, *11*, 885–896. [CrossRef]
213. Kahler, C.M.; Martin, L.E.; Shih, G.C.; Rahman, M.M.; Carlson, R.W.; Stephens, D.S. The (alpha2->8)-linked polysialic acid capsule and lipooligosaccharide structure both contribute to the ability of serogroup B *Neisseria meningitidis* to resist the bactericidal activity of normal human serum. *Infect. Immun.* **1998**, *66*, 5939–5947.
214. Masson, L.; Holbein, B.E. Influence of nutrient limitation and low pH on serogroup B *Neisseria meningitidis* capsular polysaccharide levels: Correlation with virulence for mice. *Infect. Immun.* **1985**, *47*, 465–471. [PubMed]
215. Vogel, U.; Frosch, M. Mechanisms of neisserial serum resistance. *Mol. Microbiol.* **1999**, *32*, 1133–1139. [CrossRef] [PubMed]
216. Vogel, U.; Weinberger, A.; Frank, R.; Muller, A.; Kohl, J.; Atkinson, J.P.; Frosch, M. Complement factor C3 deposition and serum resistance in isogenic capsule and lipooligosaccharide sialic acid mutants of serogroup B *Neisseria meningitidis*. *Infect. Immun.* **1997**, *65*, 4022–4029. [PubMed]
217. Claus, H.; Maiden, M.C.; Maag, R.; Frosch, M.; Vogel, U. Many carried meningococci lack the genes required for capsule synthesis and transport. *Microbiology* **2002**, *148*, 1813–1819. [CrossRef] [PubMed]
218. Claus, H.; Maiden, M.C.; Wilson, D.J.; McCarthy, N.D.; Jolley, K.A.; Urwin, R.; Hessler, F.; Frosch, M.; Vogel, U. Genetic analysis of meningococci carried by children and young adults. *J. Infect. Dis.* **2005**, *191*, 1263–1271. [CrossRef]
219. Jolley, K.A.; Kalmusova, J.; Feil, E.J.; Gupta, S.; Musilek, M.; Kriz, P.; Maiden, M.C. Carried meningococci in the Czech Republic: A diverse recombining population. *J. Clin. Microbiol.* **2000**, *38*, 4492–4498. [CrossRef]
220. Yazdankhah, S.P.; Kriz, P.; Tzanakaki, G.; Kremastinou, J.; Kalmusova, J.; Musilek, M.; Alvestad, T.; Jolley, K.A.; Wilson, D.J.; McCarthy, N.D.; et al. Distribution of serogroups and genotypes among disease-associated and carried isolates of *Neisseria meningitidis* from the Czech Republic, Greece, and Norway. *J. Clin. Microbiol.* **2004**, *42*, 5146–5153. [CrossRef]
221. Ng, L.K.; Martin, I.E. The laboratory diagnosis of *Neisseria gonorrhoeae*. *Can. J. Infect. Dis. Med. Microbiol.* **2005**, *16*, 15–25. [CrossRef]
222. Perrin, A.; Bonacorsi, S.; Carbonnelle, E.; Talibi, D.; Dessen, P.; Nassif, X.; Tinsley, C. Comparative genomics identifies the genetic islands that distinguish *Neisseria meningitidis*, the agent of cerebrospinal meningitis, from other *Neisseria* species. *Infect. Immun.* **2002**, *70*, 7063–7072. [CrossRef]
223. Chugh, K.; Bhalla, C.K.; Joshi, K.K. Meningococcal brain abscess and meningitis in a neonate. *Pediatr. Infect. Dis. J.* **1988**, *7*, 136–137. [CrossRef]
224. Herbert, D.A.; Ruskin, J. Are the "nonpathogenic" Neisseriae pathogenic? *Am. J. Clin. Pathol.* **1981**, *75*, 739–743. [CrossRef] [PubMed]
225. Kim, W.J.; Higashi, D.; Goytia, M.; Rendon, M.A.; Pilligua-Lucas, M.; Bronnimann, M.; McLean, J.A.; Duncan, J.; Trees, D.; Jerse, A.E.; et al. Commensal *Neisseria* Kill *Neisseria gonorrhoeae* through a DNA-Dependent Mechanism. *Cell Host Microbe* **2019**, *26*, 228–239.e8. [CrossRef] [PubMed]
226. Coulter, C.B. Gram-negative micrococcus causing fatal endocarditis. *Proc. N. Y. Pathol. Soc.* **1915**, *15*, 7–12.
227. Wilson, W.J. A contribution to the bacteriology of cerebrospinal meningitis. *Lancet* **1908**, *1*, 1686–1687. [CrossRef]
228. Brorson, J.E.; Axelsson, A.; Holm, S.E. Studies on *Branhamella catarrhalis* (*Neisseria catarrhalis*) with special reference to maxillary sinusitis. *Scand. J. Infect. Dis.* **1976**, *8*, 151–155. [CrossRef]
229. Coffey, J.D., Jr.; Martin, A.D.; Booth, H.N. *Neisseria catarrhalis* in exudate otitis media. *Arch. Otolaryngol.* **1967**, *86*, 403–406. [CrossRef]
230. Lee, W.S.; Fordham, T.; Alban, J. Otitis media caused by beta-lactamase-producing *Branhamella* (*Neisseria*) *catarrhalis*. *J. Clin. Microbiol.* **1981**, *13*, 222–223.
231. Schalen, L.; Christensen, P.; Kamme, C.; Miorner, H.; Pettersson, K.I.; Schalen, C. High isolation rate of *Branhamella catarrhalis* from the nasopharynx in adults with acute laryngitis. *Scand. J. Infect. Dis.* **1980**, *12*, 277–280. [CrossRef]
232. Johnson, M.A.; Drew, W.L.; Roberts, M. *Branhamella* (*Neisseria*) *catarrhalis*—A lower respiratory tract pathogen? *J. Clin. Microbiol.* **1981**, *13*, 1066–1069.

233. McNeely, D.J.; Kitchens, C.S.; Kluge, R.M. Fatal *Neisseria (Branhamella) catarrhalis* pneumonia in an immunodeficient host. *Am. Rev. Respir. Dis.* **1976**, *114*, 399–402. [CrossRef]
234. Srinivasan, G.; Raff, M.J.; Templeton, W.C.; Givens, S.J.; Graves, R.C.; Melo, J.C. *Branhamella catarrhalis* pneumonia: Report of two cases and review of the literature. *Am. Rev. Respir. Dis.* **1981**, *123*, 553–555. [CrossRef] [PubMed]
235. Ninane, G.; Joly, J.; Piot, P.; Kraytman, M. *Branhamella (Neisseria) catarrhalis* as pathogen. *Lancet* **1977**, *2*, 149. [CrossRef]
236. Ninane, G.; Joly, J.; Kraytman, M. Bronchopulmonary infection due to *Branhamella catarrhalis*: 11 cases assessed by transtracheal puncture. *Br. Med. J.* **1978**, *1*, 276–278. [CrossRef] [PubMed]
237. Ninane, G.; Joly, J.; Kraytman, M.; Piot, P. Bronchopulmonary infection due to beta-lactamase-producing *Branhamella catarrhalis* treated with amoxycillin/clavulanic-acid. *Lancet* **1978**, *2*, 257. [CrossRef]
238. Percival, A.; Corkill, J.E.; Rowlands, J.; Sykes, R.B. Pathogenicity of and beta-lactamase production by *Branhamella (Neisseria) catarrhalis*. *Lancet* **1977**, *2*, 1175. [CrossRef]
239. Verma, R.; Sood, S. Gonorrhoea diagnostics: An update. *Indian J. Med. Microbiol.* **2016**, *34*, 139–145. [CrossRef]
240. Graber, C.D.; Scott, R.C.; Dunkelberg, W.E., Jr.; Dirks, K.R. Isolation of *Neisseria catarrhalis* from three patients with urethritis and a clinical syndrome resembling gonorrhea. *Am. J. Clin. Pathol.* **1963**, *39*, 360–363. [CrossRef]
241. McCague, J.J.; McCague, N.J.; Altman, C.C. *Neisseria catarrhalis* urethritis: A case report. *J. Urol.* **1976**, *115*, 471. [CrossRef]
242. Blackwell, C.; Young, H.; Bain, S.S. Isolation of *Neisseria meningitidis* and *Neisseria catarrhalis* from the genitourinary tract and anal canal. *Br. J. Vener. Dis.* **1978**, *54*, 41–44. [CrossRef]
243. Rosenstein, N.E.; Perkins, B.A.; Stephens, D.S.; Popovic, T.; Hughes, J.M. Meningococcal disease. *N. Engl. J. Med.* **2001**, *344*, 1378–1388. [CrossRef]
244. Lee, T.J.; Utsinger, P.D.; Snyderman, R.; Yount, W.J.; Sparling, P.F. Familial deficiency of the seventh component of complement associated with recurrent bacteremic infections due to *Neisseria*. *J. Infect. Dis.* **1978**, *138*, 359–368. [CrossRef] [PubMed]
245. Palmer, A.; Criss, A.K. Gonococcal Defenses against Antimicrobial Activities of Neutrophils. *Trends Microbiol.* **2018**, *26*, 1022–1034. [CrossRef] [PubMed]
246. Escobar, A.; Rodas, P.I.; Acuna-Castillo, C. Macrophage-*Neisseria gonorrhoeae* Interactions: A Better Understanding of Pathogen Mechanisms of Immunomodulation. *Front. Immunol.* **2018**, *9*, 3044. [CrossRef] [PubMed]
247. Nadel, S. Treatment of Meningococcal Disease. *J. Adolesc. Health* **2016**, *59*, S21–S28. [CrossRef] [PubMed]
248. Feldman, H.A. Meningococcus and gonococcus: Never the Twain—Well, hardly ever. *N. Engl. J. Med.* **1971**, *285*, 518–520. [CrossRef] [PubMed]
249. Hill, D.J.; Virji, M. Meningococcal ligands and molecular targets of the host. *Methods Mol. Biol.* **2012**, *799*, 143–152. [CrossRef]
250. Meyer, T.F. Pathogenic neisseriae: Complexity of pathogen-host cell interplay. *Clin. Infect. Dis.* **1999**, *28*, 433–441. [CrossRef]
251. Naumann, M.; Rudel, T.; Meyer, T.F. Host cell interactions and signalling with *Neisseria gonorrhoeae*. *Curr. Opin. Microbiol.* **1999**, *2*, 62–70. [CrossRef]
252. Plant, L.; Jonsson, A.B. Contacting the host: Insights and implications of pathogenic *Neisseria* cell interactions. *Scand. J. Infect. Dis.* **2003**, *35*, 608–613. [CrossRef]
253. Apicella, M.A.; Shao, J.; Neil, R.B. Methods for studying *Neisseria meningitidis* biofilms. *Methods Mol. Biol.* **2012**, *799*, 169–184. [CrossRef]
254. Hall-Stoodley, L.; Costerton, J.W.; Stoodley, P. Bacterial biofilms: From the natural environment to infectious diseases. *Nat. Rev. Microbiol.* **2004**, *2*, 95–108. [CrossRef] [PubMed]
255. Carbonnelle, E.; Hill, D.J.; Morand, P.; Griffiths, N.J.; Bourdoulous, S.; Murillo, I.; Nassif, X.; Virji, M. Meningococcal interactions with the host. *Vaccine* **2009**, *27* (Suppl. 2), B78–B89. [CrossRef]
256. Hill, D.J.; Griffiths, N.J.; Borodina, E.; Virji, M. Cellular and molecular biology of *Neisseria meningitidis* colonization and invasive disease. *Clin. Sci. (Lond.)* **2010**, *118*, 547–564. [CrossRef] [PubMed]
257. Hung, M.C.; Christodoulides, M. The biology of *Neisseria* adhesins. *Biology (Basel)* **2013**, *2*, 1054–1109. [CrossRef] [PubMed]

258. Merz, A.J.; So, M. Interactions of pathogenic Neisseriae with epithelial cell membranes. *Annu. Rev. Cell Dev. Biol.* **2000**, *16*, 423–457. [CrossRef]
259. Virji, M. Pathogenic Neisseriae: Surface modulation, pathogenesis and infection control. *Nat. Rev. Microbiol.* **2009**, *7*, 274–286. [CrossRef]
260. Strom, M.S.; Lory, S. Structure-function and biogenesis of the type IV pili. *Annu. Rev. Microbiol.* **1993**, *47*, 565–596. [CrossRef]
261. Virji, M.; Heckels, J.E. Antigenic cross-reactivity of *Neisseria* pili: Investigations with type- and species-specific monoclonal antibodies. *J. Gen. Microbiol.* **1983**, *129*, 2761–2768. [CrossRef]
262. Aho, E.L.; Keating, A.M.; McGillivray, S.M. A comparative analysis of pilin genes from pathogenic and nonpathogenic *Neisseria* species. *Microb. Pathog.* **2000**, *28*, 81–88. [CrossRef]
263. Zhu, P.; Morelli, G.; Achtman, M. The *opcA* and (psi)*opcB* regions in *Neisseria*: Genes, pseudogenes, deletions, insertion elements and DNA islands. *Mol. Microbiol.* **1999**, *33*, 635–650. [CrossRef]
264. Zhu, P.; Klutch, M.J.; Derrick, J.P.; Prince, S.M.; Tsang, R.S.; Tsai, C.M. Identification of *opcA* gene in *Neisseria polysaccharea*: Interspecies diversity of Opc protein family. *Gene* **2003**, *307*, 31–40. [CrossRef]
265. Swanson, J. Studies on gonococcus infection. XIV. Cell wall protein differences among color/opacity colony variants of *Neisseria gonorrhoeae*. *Infect. Immun.* **1978**, *21*, 292–302. [PubMed]
266. Sadarangani, M.; Hoe, C.J.; Makepeace, K.; van der Ley, P.; Pollard, A.J. Phase variation of Opa proteins of *Neisseria meningitidis* and the effects of bacterial transformation. *J. Biosci.* **2016**, *41*, 13–19. [CrossRef] [PubMed]
267. Toleman, M.; Aho, E.; Virji, M. Expression of pathogen-like Opa adhesins in commensal *Neisseria*: Genetic and functional analysis. *Cell Microbiol.* **2001**, *3*, 33–44. [CrossRef] [PubMed]
268. Hadi, H.A.; Wooldridge, K.G.; Robinson, K.; Ala'Aldeen, D.A. Identification and characterization of App: An immunogenic autotransporter protein of *Neisseria meningitidis*. *Mol. Microbiol.* **2001**, *41*, 611–623. [CrossRef]
269. Serruto, D.; Adu-Bobie, J.; Scarselli, M.; Veggi, D.; Pizza, M.; Rappuoli, R.; Arico, B. *Neisseria meningitidis* App, a new adhesin with autocatalytic serine protease activity. *Mol. Microbiol.* **2003**, *48*, 323–334. [CrossRef]
270. Comanducci, M.; Bambini, S.; Caugant, D.A.; Mora, M.; Brunelli, B.; Capecchi, B.; Ciucchi, L.; Rappuoli, R.; Pizza, M. NadA diversity and carriage in *Neisseria meningitidis*. *Infect. Immun.* **2004**, *72*, 4217–4223. [CrossRef]
271. Scarselli, M.; Serruto, D.; Montanari, P.; Capecchi, B.; Adu-Bobie, J.; Veggi, D.; Rappuoli, R.; Pizza, M.; Arico, B. *Neisseria meningitidis* NhhA is a multifunctional trimeric autotransporter adhesin. *Mol. Microbiol.* **2006**, *61*, 631–644. [CrossRef]
272. Arking, D.; Tong, Y.; Stein, D.C. Analysis of lipooligosaccharide biosynthesis in the Neisseriaceae. *J. Bacteriol.* **2001**, *183*, 934–941. [CrossRef]
273. Zhu, P.; Klutch, M.J.; Bash, M.C.; Tsang, R.S.; Ng, L.K.; Tsai, C.M. Genetic diversity of three *lgt* loci for biosynthesis of lipooligosaccharide (LOS) in *Neisseria* species. *Microbiology* **2002**, *148*, 1833–1844. [CrossRef]
274. Feavers, I.M.; Maiden, M.C. A gonococcal *porA* pseudogene: Implications for understanding the evolution and pathogenicity of *Neisseria gonorrhoeae*. *Mol. Microbiol.* **1998**, *30*, 647–656. [CrossRef] [PubMed]
275. Derrick, J.P.; Urwin, R.; Suker, J.; Feavers, I.M.; Maiden, M.C. Structural and evolutionary inference from molecular variation in *Neisseria* porins. *Infect. Immun.* **1999**, *67*, 2406–2413. [PubMed]
276. Marri, P.R.; Paniscus, M.; Weyand, N.J.; Rendon, M.A.; Calton, C.M.; Hernandez, D.R.; Higashi, D.L.; Sodergren, E.; Weinstock, G.M.; Rounsley, S.D.; et al. Genome sequencing reveals widespread virulence gene exchange among human *Neisseria* species. *PLoS ONE* **2010**, *5*, e11835. [CrossRef] [PubMed]
277. Snyder, L.A.; Saunders, N.J. The majority of genes in the pathogenic *Neisseria* species are present in non-pathogenic *Neisseria lactamica*, including those designated as 'virulence genes'. *BMC Genom.* **2006**, *7*, 128. [CrossRef] [PubMed]
278. Jordan, P.W.; Snyder, L.A.; Saunders, N.J. Strain-specific differences in *Neisseria gonorrhoeae* associated with the phase variable gene repertoire. *BMC Microbiol.* **2005**, *5*, 21. [CrossRef] [PubMed]
279. Klughammer, J.; Dittrich, M.; Blom, J.; Mitesser, V.; Vogel, U.; Frosch, M.; Goesmann, A.; Muller, T.; Schoen, C. Comparative Genome Sequencing Reveals Within-Host Genetic Changes in *Neisseria meningitidis* during Invasive Disease. *PLoS ONE* **2017**, *12*, e0169892. [CrossRef]

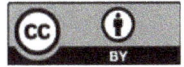

© 2019 by the authors. Licensee MDPI, Basel, Switzerland. This article is an open access article distributed under the terms and conditions of the Creative Commons Attribution (CC BY) license (http://creativecommons.org/licenses/by/4.0/).

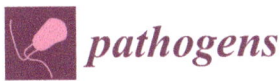

Brief Report

Commensal *Neisseria* Are Shared between Sexual Partners: Implications for Gonococcal and Meningococcal Antimicrobial Resistance

Christophe Van Dijck [1], Jolein G. E. Laumen [1], Sheeba S. Manoharan-Basil [1] and Chris Kenyon [1,2,*]

1. Department of Clinical Sciences, Institute of Tropical Medicine Antwerp, 2000 Antwerp, Belgium; cvandijck@itg.be (C.V.D.)
2. Department of Medicine, University of Cape Town, Cape Town 7700, South Africa
* Correspondence: ckenyon@itg.be

Received: 22 February 2020; Accepted: 16 March 2020; Published: 19 March 2020

Abstract: Antimicrobial resistance in pathogenic *Neisseria* parallels reduced antimicrobial susceptibility in commensal *Neisseria* in certain populations, like men who have sex with men (MSM). Although this reduced susceptibility can be a consequence of frequent antimicrobial exposure at the individual level, we hypothesized that commensal *Neisseria* are transmitted between sexual partners. We used data from a 2014 microbiome study in which saliva and tongue swabs were taken from 21 couples (42 individuals). Samples were analyzed using 16S rRNA gene sequencing. We compared intimate partners with unrelated individuals and found that the oral *Neisseria* communities of intimate partners were more similar than those of unrelated individuals (average Morisita–Horn dissimilarity index for saliva samples: 0.54 versus 0.71, respectively ($p = 0.005$); and for tongue swabs: 0.42 versus 0.63, respectively ($p = 0.006$)). This similarity presumably results from transmission of oral *Neisseria* through intimate kissing. This finding suggests that intensive gonorrhea screening in MSM may, via increased antimicrobial exposure, promote, rather than prevent, the emergence and spread of antimicrobial resistance in *Neisseria*. Non-antibiotic strategies such as vaccines and oral antiseptics could prove more sustainable options to reduce gonococcal prevalence.

Keywords: commensal; *Neisseria*; gonorrhea; *meningitidis*; kissing; sharing; microbiome; transmission; antimicrobial resistance

1. Introduction

Neisseria gonorrhoeae has rapidly acquired resistance to all antimicrobials used to treat it, and there is a real risk that it may be untreatable in the near future [1]. It is increasingly appreciated that a key way it acquires this antimicrobial resistance (AMR) is via taking up resistance genes from oropharyngeal commensal *Neisseria*. The genus *Neisseria* is one of the three most abundant phyla in the human oral microbiome [2], with almost all individuals being colonized with at least one *Neisseria* species [3]. This high prevalence, in combination with extensive antimicrobial exposure, is thought to explain the extensive AMR in commensal *Neisseria* that has been found in certain populations, like cohorts of men who have sex with men (MSM) [4] and that has played an important role in the genesis of AMR in *N. gonorrhoeae* [5].

Epidemiological and modeling studies evaluating the emergence of AMR in *N. gonorrhoeae* have typically included the sexual transmission of resistant gonococci but not commensal *Neisseria* [6,7]. If resistant commensal *Neisseria* were also sexually transmitted, this would be important to take into consideration. This would be particularly important if these commensals could be transferred via highly prevalent activities such as tongue kissing. Transfer via kissing would diminish the likelihood that traditional gonorrhea control measures would work to control the genesis and spread of gonococcal AMR. In certain instances, they may even be counterproductive. Several authors have, for example, suggested that because pharyngeal gonorrhea plays such an important role in the emergence of AMR (via horizontal gene transfer from commensals), intensive screening and treatment of pharyngeal gonorrhea in MSM should be advocated [1]. This strategy has been shown to result in extremely high antimicrobial exposure with a resultant high probability of inducing AMR in commensal *Neisseria* [8]. If these resistant *Neisseria* were then transferred via kissing and these resulted in AMR in *N. gonorrhoeae*, then intensive screening may indirectly increase rather than decrease the probability of gonococcal AMR emergence.

Concerns around the transmission of commensal *Neisseria* via kissing have emerged following increasing evidence of this mode of transmission for related bacteria. Several studies have found that kissing is a risk factor for meningococcal disease [9–11] or carriage [12–15] among students. Likewise, *N. gonorrhoeae* can be readily cultured from saliva [16–18], saliva use as a lubricant is a risk factor for rectal gonorrhea [19], kissing [20–22] as well as having a main partner with pharyngeal gonorrhea [23] may be risk factors for pharyngeal gonorrhea and a mathematical transmission model showed that oro–oral transmission is essential to generate the actual prevalence of gonorrhea among MSM [6].

Furthermore, a number of studies have found that the oral microbiome is shared between household members [24,25]. An important study by Kort et al. in 2014 demonstrated that intimate partners share a similar oral microbiome and that the degree of similarity of the salivary microbiota correlates with the kissing-frequency in the past weeks and with the time since the last kiss [26]. They calculated that an intimate kiss of 10 seconds leads to an average transfer of 10^8 bacteria from one partner to another [26].

These considerations led us to hypothesize that commensal *Neisseria* are transmitted between sexual partners. To test this hypothesis, we performed a secondary analysis of the study by Kort et al. We found that kissing partners shared more similar *Neisseria* communities than unrelated individuals.

2. Results

The dataset provided by Kort et al. [26] consisted of tongue and salivary microbiota samples taken from 21 couples visiting a Zoo in 2012. We compared the results from the entire range of 3000 operational taxonomic units (OTUs) with those from the 66 OTUs which represent members of the genus *Neisseria*. We found that pairwise comparison of samples using the Morisita–Horn dissimilarity index (MHi) did not differ significantly for analyses based on the entire versus the restricted dataset. Based on *Neisseria*-related OTUs we found the following:

1. A high pairwise similarity (an MHi value close to zero) between duplicate samples of an individual's tongue surface (MHi 0.17) and saliva (MHi 0.28) indicated that sampling was reproducible at the level of the genus *Neisseria* (Figure 1).
2. Partners' oral *Neisseria* communities sampled after a 10-second kiss were not more similar than before the kiss (saliva: average MHi 0.55 before versus 0.53 after, $p = 0.704$; surface of the tongue: average MHi 0.39 before versus 0.45 after, $p = 0.597$; Figure 1). Therefore, samples before and after kissing were combined in the subsequent analyses.
3. Partners' oral *Neisseria* communities were more similar compared to unrelated individuals. This was found for saliva (average MHi 0.54 versus 0.71, respectively, $p = 0.005$) and for samples of the tongue surface (average MHi 0.42 versus 0.63, respectively, $p = 0.006$; Figure 1).

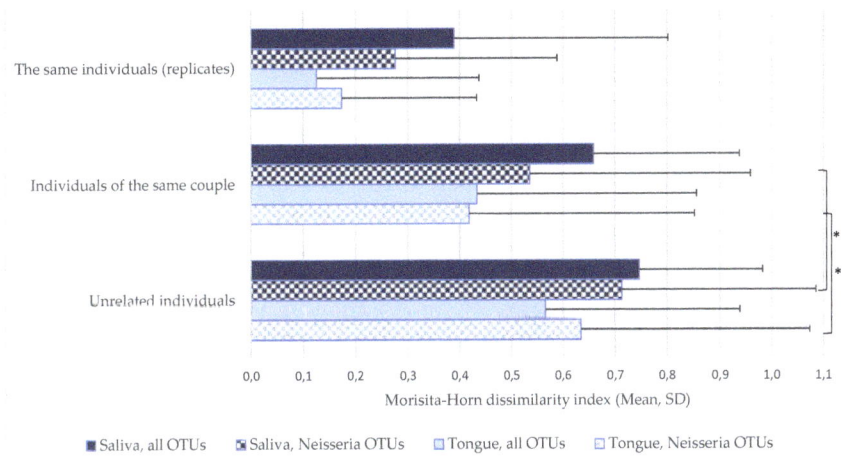

Figure 1. Morisita–Horn dissimilarity indices of samples from the same individuals, intimate partners and unrelated individuals. An index of 0 represents complete similarity whereas an index of 1 means complete dissimilarity. Each bar shows the average Morisita–Horn index, whiskers indicate standard deviations, * $p < 0.01$.

3. Discussion

Although it was already known that household members and intimate partners share oral commensal microbiota [24–26], the current analysis demonstrates that intimate partners also share similar commensal *Neisseria*. This is a logical, yet important finding, as commensal *Neisseria* are known to harbor several AMR determinants [27] that are a frequent source of AMR for pathogenic *Neisseria* [4,28,29].

Sharing of commensal *Neisseria* via this and other modalities may, therefore, explain the high prevalence of antimicrobial resistant commensal *Neisseria* in certain groups of patients. A study from Japan in 2005–2006, reported the antimicrobial susceptibility of 45 oropharyngeal *Neisseria subflava* isolates from men with urethritis and female commercial sex workers. The majority of isolates had reduced susceptibility to penicillin, tetracycline and ciprofloxacin [30]. Another study in Vietnam in 2016–2017 investigated 265 *Neisseria* isolates from 207 MSM, including 9 gonococci and 13 meningococci. Ten different *Neisseria* species were identified. Twenty-eight percent of samples had reduced susceptibility to ceftriaxone (minimum inhibitory concentration ≥ 0.125 mg/L) [4]. The reason for the high prevalence of commensal *Neisseria* with reduced antimicrobial susceptibility in these groups of patients presumably parallels the one proposed for gonorrhea: repeated cycles of reinfection/recolonization and antimicrobial exposure in individuals within a highly connected transmission-network [31].

In addition, since the pharynx is the predominant reservoir of nonpathogenic *Neisseria* in humans, it is probable that *Neisseria* are transmitted between partners by transfer of saliva, either directly (by intimate kissing or through aerosolized droplets), or indirectly (e.g., through shared fomites). The scarcity of nonpathogenic *Neisseria* within other bodily niches makes it unlikely that the skin, genital or anorectal site act as an intermediate in this transfer process. As already noted, different types of evidence suggest that pathogenic *Neisseria* species can be transmitted by kissing [6,9–23]. Our findings support to the idea that the genus *Neisseria* can be transmitted by kissing.

The limitations of this study include the following. First, the fact that partners share certain microbiota does not provide direct evidence of transmission between them. Intimate kissing may be one explanation, but we have not explored alternative means of transmission. Potential mediators of transmission could be via fomites or animals (such as pets), or influences on the oral microbiota by environmental factors, common diet or simultaneous exposure to pathogens, toxins, mouthwashes or antimicrobials [32]. Second, identification of the oral microbiota in this study was based on the amplification of hypervariable regions V5–V7 of the 16S rRNA gene. This does not allow for the accurate identification of microbiota at the species level, nor does it provide information concerning antimicrobial susceptibility of the microbiota involved. Still, it seems reasonable to infer that sharing of specific OTUs represents sharing of a specific subset of bacterial genomes and, thus, AMR determinants within these bacteria.

The significance of this study lies in its relevance for preventing the further emergence of AMR in *N. gonorrhoeae* and *N. meningitidis*. If commensal *Neisseria* can be spread by common-place activities such as kissing, then this increases the probability that intensive gonorrhea screening in high prevalence populations such as MSM will, via increased antimicrobial exposure, promote, rather than retard, the emergence of AMR in *Neisseria*. Certain groups of at-risk populations are frequently exposed to antibiotics to treat symptomatic sexually transmitted infections. Treatment of asymptomatic cases increases this exposure even more. As most cases of anorectal and pharyngeal gonorrhea are asymptomatic, regular screening of asymptomatic patients results in a much higher number of diagnosed infections and, thus, a substantial increase in antibiotic exposure [33]. Currently, several guidelines recommend regular gonorrhea screening among MSM at high risk of infection [34,35]. The idea behind this is that treatment of all cases of gonorrhea in a population would eventually lead to a reduction (or eradication) of the pathogen from that population. There is, however, very little empirical evidence that supports this hypothesis [36]. On the other hand, increased antimicrobial exposure has been linked to AMR in gonorrhea [37,38]. This, together with the finding from the current study that *Neisseria* (including AMR determinants) may be transmitted to other individuals within a network via kissing, provides another pathway for the dissemination of AMR. Intensive screening and treatment of all positives may have a profound impact on the prevalence of AMR in commensal *Neisseria*, which could then be rapidly spread between individuals by kissing. A more prudent approach to preventing the emergence of AMR would be to reduce antimicrobial exposure as far as possible. This could include reduced screening and using non-antibiotic strategies such as vaccines and oral antiseptics to reduce gonococcal prevalence [39,40].

4. Materials and Methods

4.1. Sample Collection and Processing

In the study by Kort et al., samples were collected from 42 individuals (21 couples) visiting a Zoo in the Netherlands in 2014. A swab was taken from the anterior dorsal surface of the tongue and saliva was collected in a sterile 15 mL tube. Each participant was sampled before and after an intimate kiss of 10 s. Three couples were sampled in duplicate in order to assess reproducibility. Samples were stored at −80 °C until further processing. After DNA extraction, quantitative 16S rRNA PCR was used to generate an amplicon library based on the 16S variable regions V5-V7. Aligned 16S rRNA sequences were clustered into OTUs, defined by 97% sequence similarity. The RDP Naive Bayesian Classifier and the SILVA reference database (release 119) were used for taxonomic classification. The full study protocol is described in the original paper [26].

4.2. Availability of Data and Materials

The dataset supporting the conclusions of this article is available as a supplementary file to the paper by Kort et al. [26] For the *Neisseria*-specific analysis, the dataset was restricted to only those 66 OTUs representing members of the genus *Neisseria*.

4.3. Assessment of Community Similarity

Similarity of tongue and salivary microbiota (β-diversity) was determined by calculating pairwise distances with the Morisita–Horn dissimilarity index [41] using R version 3.6.1. A value of zero on this index represents complete similarity, whereas a value of one means complete dissimilarity.

4.4. Statistical Analysis

The non-parametric Wilcoxon rank-sum test in R was used to calculate the *p*-values for selected paired differences of data. Data were visualized using Microsoft Excel.

4.5. Ethics Approval and Consent to Participate

Not applicable.

Author Contributions: Conceptualization, C.V.D., J.G.E.L. and C.K.; methodology, C.V.D. and C.K.; formal analysis, C.V.D.; writing—original draft preparation, C.V.D.; writing—review and editing, C.V.D., J.G.E.L., S.S.M.-B. and C.K.; visualization, C.V.D. All authors have read and agreed to the published version of the manuscript.

Funding: This research received no external funding.

Conflicts of Interest: The authors declare no conflict of interest.

Abbreviations

The following abbreviations are used in this manuscript:
AMR   antimicrobial resistance
MSM   men who have sex with men
OTU   operational taxonomic unit
MHi   Morisita–Horn index

References

1. Wi, T.; Lahra, M.M.; Ndowa, F.; Bala, M.; Dillon, J.A.R.; Ramon-Pardo, P.; Eremin, S.R.; Bolan, G.; Unemo, M. Antimicrobial resistance in Neisseria gonorrhoeae: Global surveillance and a call for international collaborative action. *PLoS Med.* **2017**, *14*, e1002344. [CrossRef]
2. Verma, D.; Garg, P.K.; Dubey, A.K. Insights into the human oral microbiome. *Arch. Microbiol.* **2018**, *200*, 525–540. [CrossRef]
3. Sâez, J.A.; Carmen, N.; Vinde, M.A. Multicolonization of human nasopharynx due to Neisseria spp. *Int. Microbiol.* **1998**, *1*, 59–63. [CrossRef]
4. Dong, H.V.; Pham, L.Q.; Nguyen, H.T.; Nguyen, M.X.B.; Nguyen, T.V.; May, F.; Le, G.M.; Klausner, J.D. Decreased Cephalosporin Susceptibility of Oropharyngeal Neisseria Species in Antibiotic-using Men Who Have Sex With Men in Hanoi, Vietnam. *Clin. Infect. Dis.* **2019**. [CrossRef]
5. Lewis, D.A. The role of core groups in the emergence and dissemination of antimicrobial-resistant N gonorrhoeae. *Sex. Transm. Infect.* **2013**, *89*. [CrossRef]
6. Zhang, L.; Regan, D.G.; Chow, E.P.; Gambhir, M.; Cornelisse, V.; Grulich, A.; Ong, J.; Lewis, D.A.; Hocking, J.; Fairley, C.K. Neisseria gonorrhoeae Transmission among Men Who Have Sex with Men: An Anatomical Site-Specific Mathematical Model Evaluating the Potential Preventive Impact of Mouthwash. *Sex. Transm. Dis.* **2017**, *44*, 586–592. [CrossRef]
7. Fairley, C.K.; Cornelisse, V.J.; Hocking, J.S.; Chow, E.P.F. Models of gonorrhoea transmission from the mouth and saliva. *Lancet Infect. Dis.* **2019**, 1–7. [CrossRef]
8. Kenyon, C. We need to consider collateral damage to resistomes when we decide how frequently to screen for chlamydia/gonorrhoea in PrEP cohorts. *AIDS* **2019**, *33*, 155–157. [CrossRef]
9. Tully, J.; Viner, R.M.; Coen, P.G.; Stuart, J.M.; Zambon, M.; Peckham, C.; Booth, C.; Klein, N.; Kaczmarski, E.; Booy, R. Risk and protective factors for meningococcal disease in adolescents: Matched cohort study. *Br. Med. J.* **2006**, *332*, 445–448. [CrossRef]

10. Mandal, S.; Wu, H.M.; MacNeil, J.R.; Machesky, K.; Garcia, J.; Plikaytis, B.D.; Quinn, K.; King, L.; Schmink, S.E.; Wang, X.; et al. Prolonged university outbreak of meningococcal disease associated with a serogroup B strain rarely seen in the United States. *Clin. Infect. Dis.* **2013**, *57*, 344–348. [CrossRef]
11. Stanwell-Smith, R.E.; Stuart, J.M.; Hughes, A.O.; Robinson, P.; Griffin, M.B.; Cartwright, K. Smoking, the environment and meningococcal disease: A case control study. *Epidemiol. Infect.* **1994**, *112*, 315–328. [CrossRef]
12. McMillan, M.; Walters, L.; Mark, T.; Lawrence, A.; Leong, L.E.; Sullivan, T.; Rogers, G.B.; Andrews, R.M.; Marshall, H.S. B Part of It study: A longitudinal study to assess carriage of Neisseria meningitidis in first year university students in South Australia. *Hum. Vaccines Immunother.* **2019**, *15*, 987–994. [CrossRef]
13. Van Ravenhorst, M.B.; Bijlsma, M.W.; van Houten, M.A.; Struben, V.M.; Anderson, A.S.; Eiden, J.; Hao, L.; Jansen, K.U.; Jones, H.; Kitchin, N.; et al. Meningococcal carriage in Dutch adolescents and young adults; a cross-sectional and longitudinal cohort study. *Clin. Microbiol. Infect.* **2017**, *23*, 573.e1–573.e7. [CrossRef]
14. Neal, K.R.; Nguyen-Van-Tam, J.S.; Jeffrey, N.; Slack, R.C.; Madeley, R.J.; Ait-Tahar, K.; Job, K.; Wale, M.C.; Ala'aldeen, D.A. Changing carriage rate of Neisseria meningitidis among university students during the first week of term: Cross sectional study. *Bmj* **2000**, *320*, 846–849. [CrossRef]
15. Marshall, H.S.; McMillan, M.; Koehler, A.; Lawrence, A.; Sullivan, T.; MacLennan, J.M.; Maiden, M.C.; Ladhani, S.N.; Ramsay, M.; Trotter, C.; et al. Impact of meningococcal B vaccine on meningococcal carriage in adolescents. *N. Engl. J. Med.* **2019**, 318–327, in Press. [CrossRef]
16. Hallqvist, L.; Lindgren, S. Gonorrhoea of the throat at a venereological clinic incidence and results of treatment. *Sex. Transm. Infect.* **1975**, *51*, 395–397. [CrossRef]
17. Hutt, D.M.; Judson, F.N. Epidemiology and treatment of oropharyngeal gonorrhea. *Ann. Intern. Med.* **1986**, *104*, 655–658. [CrossRef]
18. Chow, E.P.; Lee, D.; Tabrizi, S.N.; Phillips, S.; Snow, A.; Cook, S.; Howden, B.P.; Petalotis, I.; Bradshaw, C.S.; Chen, M.Y.; et al. Detection of Neisseria gonorrhoeae in the pharynx and saliva: Implications for gonorrhoea transmission. *Sex. Transm. Infect.* **2016**, *92*, 347–349. [CrossRef]
19. Chow, E.P.; Cornelisse, V.J.; Read, T.R.; Lee, D.; Walker, S.; Hocking, J.S.; Chen, M.Y.; Bradshaw, C.S.; Fairley, C.K. Saliva use as a lubricant for anal sex is a risk factor for rectal gonorrhoea among men who have sex with men, a new public health message: A cross-sectional survey. *Sex. Transm. Infect.* **2016**. [CrossRef]
20. Templeton, D.J.; Jin, F.; McNally, L.P.; Imrie, J.C.; Prestage, G.P.; Donovan, B.; Cunningham, P.H.; Kaldor, J.M.; Kippax, S.; Grulich, A.E. Prevalence, incidence and risk factors for pharyngeal gonorrhoea in a community-based HIV-negative cohort of homosexual men in Sydney, Australia. *Sex. Transm. Infect.* **2010**, *86*, 90–96. [CrossRef]
21. Cornelisse, V.J.; Walker, S.; Phillips, T.; Hocking, J.S.; Bradshaw, C.S.; Lewis, D.A.; Prestage, G.P.; Grulich, A.E.; Fairley, C.K.; Chow, E.P. Risk factors for oropharyngeal gonorrhoea in men who have sex with men: An age-matched case-control study. *Sex. Transm. Infect.* **2018**, *94*, 359–364. [CrossRef]
22. Chow, E.P.F.; Cornelisse, V.J.; Williamson, D.A.; Priest, D.; Hocking, J.S.; Bradshaw, C.S.; Read, T.R.H.; Chen, M.Y.; Howden, B.P.; Fairley, C.K. Kissing may be an important and neglected risk factor for oropharyngeal gonorrhoea: A cross-sectional study in men who have sex with men. *Sex. Transm. Infect.* **2019**, *95*. [CrossRef]
23. Cornelisse, V.J.; Zhang, L.; Law, M.; Chen, M.Y.; Bradshaw, C.S.; Bellhouse, C.; Fairley, C.K.; Chow, E.P. Concordance of gonorrhoea of the rectum, pharynx and urethra in same-sex male partnerships attending a sexual health service in Melbourne, Australia. *BMC Infect. Dis.* **2018**, *18*. [CrossRef]
24. Song, J.; Lauber, C.; Costello, E.K.; Lozupone, C.A.; Humphrey, G.; Berg-Lyons, D.; Caporaso, J.G.; Knights, D.; Clemente, J.C.; Nakielny, S.; et al. Cohabiting family members share microbiota with one another and with their dogs. *eLife* **2013**, *2013*, 1–22. [CrossRef]
25. Abeles, S.R.; Jones, M.B.; Santiago-Rodriguez, T.M.; Ly, M.; Klitgord, N.; Yooseph, S.; Nelson, K.E.; Pride, D.T. Microbial diversity in individuals and their household contacts following typical antibiotic courses. *Microbiome* **2016**, *4*, 1–12. [CrossRef]
26. Kort, R.; Caspers, M.; van de Graaf, A.; van Egmond, W.; Keijser, B.; Roeselers, G. Shaping the oral microbiota through intimate kissing. *Microbiome* **2014**, *2*, 1–8. [CrossRef]
27. Marangoni, A.; Marziali, G.; Salvo, M.; D'Antuono, A.; Gaspari, V.; Foschi, C.; Re, M.C. Mosaic structure of the penA gene in the oropharynx of men who have sex with men negative for gonorrhoea. *Int. J. STD AIDS* **2020**. [CrossRef]

28. Igawa, G.; Yamagishi, Y.; Lee, K.I.I.; Dorin, M.; Shimuta, K.; Suematsu, H.; Nakayama, S.I.I.; Mikamo, H.; Unemo, M.; Ohnishi, M.; et al. Neisseria cinerea with high ceftriaxone MIC Is a source of ceftriaxone and cefixime resistance-mediating penA sequences in Neisseria gonorrhoeae. *Antimicrob. Agents Chemother.* **2018**, *62*, 1–5. [CrossRef]
29. Wadsworth, C.B.; Arnold, B.J.; Sater, M.R.A.; Grad, Y.H. Azithromycin Resistance through Interspecific Acquisition of an Epistasis-Dependent Efflux Pump Component and Transcriptional Regulator in Neisseria gonorrhoeae. *mBio* **2018**, *9*, 1–17. [CrossRef]
30. Furuya, R.; Onoye, Y.; Kanayama, A.; Saika, T.; Iyoda, T.; Tatewaki, M.; Matsuzaki, K.; Kobayashi, I.; Tanaka, M. Antimicrobial resistance in clinical isolates of Neisseria subflava from the oral cavities of a Japanese population. *J. Infect. Chemother.* **2007**, *13*, 302–304. [CrossRef]
31. Kenyon, C.R.; Schwartz, I.S. Effects of sexual network connectivity and antimicrobial drug use on antimicrobial resistance in neisseria gonorrhoeae. *Emerg. Infect. Dis.* **2018**, *24*, 1195–1203. [CrossRef] [PubMed]
32. Trinh, P.; Zaneveld, J.R.; Safranek, S.; Rabinowitz, P.M. One Health Relationships Between Human, Animal, and Environmental Microbiomes: A Mini-Review. *Front. Public Health* **2018**, *6*, 1–9. [CrossRef] [PubMed]
33. Kenyon, C. How actively should we screen for chlamydia and gonorrhoea in MSM and other high-ST-prevalence populations as we enter the era of increasingly untreatable infections? A viewpoint. *J. Med Microbiol.* **2019**, *68*, 132–135. [CrossRef] [PubMed]
34. Tan, D.H.; Hull, M.W.; Yoong, D.; Tremblay, C.; O'Byrne, P.; Thomas, R.; Kille, J.; Baril, J.G.; Cox, J.; Giguere, P.; et al. Canadian guideline on HIV pre-exposure prophylaxis and nonoccupational postexposure prophylaxis. *CMAJ* **2017**, *189*, E1448–E1458. [CrossRef] [PubMed]
35. Australian Sexually Transmitted Infection & HIV Testing Guidelines 2019 for Asymptomatic Men Who Have Sex with Men. Available online: http://www.sti.guidelines.org.au (accessed on 18 March 2020).
36. Ridpath, A.D.; Chesson, H.; Marcus, J.L.; Kirkcaldy, R.D.; Torrone, E.A.; Aral, S.O.; Bernstein, K.T. Screening Peter to Save Paul: The Population-Level Effects of Screening Men Who Have Sex with Men for Gonorrhea and Chlamydia. *Sex. Transm. Dis.* **2018**, *45*, 623–625. [CrossRef] [PubMed]
37. Kenyon, C.; Buyze, J.; Spiteri, G.; Cole, M.J.; Unemo, M. Population-Level Antimicrobial Consumption Is Associated With Decreased Antimicrobial Susceptibility in Neisseria gonorrhoeae in 24 European Countries: An Ecological Analysis. *J. Infect. Dis.* **2019**, *8*. [CrossRef]
38. Wind, C.M.; De Vries, E.; Schim Van Der Loeff, M.F.; Van Rooijen, M.S.; Van Dam, A.P.; Demczuk, W.H.; Martin, I.; De Vries, H.J. Decreased Azithromycin Susceptibility of Neisseria gonorrhoeae Isolates in Patients Recently Treated with Azithromycin. *Clin. Infect. Dis.* **2017**, *65*, 37–45. [CrossRef]
39. Chow, E.P.; Walker, S.; Hocking, J.S.; Bradshaw, C.S.; Chen, M.Y.; Tabrizi, S.N.; Howden, B.P.; Law, M.G.; Maddaford, K.; Read, T.R.; et al. A multicentre double-blind randomised controlled trial evaluating the efficacy of daily use of antibacterial mouthwash against oropharyngeal gonorrhoea among men who have sex with men: The OMEGA (Oral Mouthwash use to Eradicate GonorrhoeA) study protocol. *BMC Infect. Dis.* **2017**, *17*, 456. [CrossRef]
40. Paynter, J.; Goodyear-Smith, F.; Morgan, J.; Saxton, P.; Black, S.; Petousis-Harris, H. Effectiveness of a group b outer membrane vesicle meningococcal vaccine in preventing hospitalization from gonorrhea in New Zealand: A retrospective cohort study. *Vaccines* **2019**, *7*, 1–11. [CrossRef]
41. Horn, H.S. Measurement of "Overlap" in Comparative Ecological Studies. *Am. Nat.* **1966**, *100*, 419–424. [CrossRef]

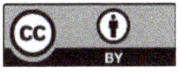

© 2020 by the authors. Licensee MDPI, Basel, Switzerland. This article is an open access article distributed under the terms and conditions of the Creative Commons Attribution (CC BY) license (http://creativecommons.org/licenses/by/4.0/).

MDPI
St. Alban-Anlage 66
4052 Basel
Switzerland
Tel. +41 61 683 77 34
Fax +41 61 302 89 18
www.mdpi.com

Pathogens Editorial Office
E-mail: pathogens@mdpi.com
www.mdpi.com/journal/pathogens

www.ingramcontent.com/pod-product-compliance
Lightning Source LLC
LaVergne TN
LVHW070544100526
838202LV00012B/373